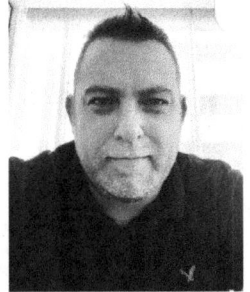

Jason Sullivan is a mental-health therapist at Kuwait Counseling Center, and the founder of Quiet Chaos. Jason is also a speaker and a writer. He has presented on student mental-health issues in a university environment at the MENASPA Conferences in Singapore and Kuwait, which is an international conference for student affairs professionals from the Middle East, North Africa, and Asia. He has also presented for the Indian Women's Association of Kuwait on addiction, as well as the Middle East Psychological Association on the physiology of anxiety disorders. He is the former director of the Counseling Center at the American University of Kuwait, 2011–2019.

Jason has a bachelor's degree in philosophy and religious studies, as well as a master's degree in mental-health counseling. He has been involved in outreach work through his Quiet Chaos campaign, as well as creating the first art and music therapy program in a university in the Middle East. Jason is a member of the American Counseling Association, Florida Crisis Response Team, and Middle East Psychological Association.

Roger Shepherd – for being the example of unwavering love and acceptance. Your friendship held me in the worst moments and encouraged me to grow with such gentleness and embrace. Words will never express the place that you have in my heart.

Dan Miller – for walking the tough journey with me and for giving me the words that I needed to hear, even though it took years for me to listen. You are, and always will be, my brother.

Dewayne Wood – for being my friend. I still hear your laugh and wise words. The world lost a great man, but you live on in the hearts of those who knew you.

Shirley Sullivan – my wife, my friend, and the person who lovingly tolerated a philosophical therapist with grace and patience. Thank you, love.

Jason R. Sullivan

QUIET CHAOS

THE LINK BETWEEN ANXIETY AND AWARENESS

AUSTIN MACAULEY PUBLISHERS™

LONDON • CAMBRIDGE • NEW YORK • SHARJAH

ISBN – 9789948340232– (Paperback)
ISBN – 9789948340225 – (E-Book)

Application Number: MC-10-01-7521972
Age Classification: E

First Published (2020)
AUSTIN MACAULEY PUBLISHERS FZE
Sharjah Publishing City
P.O Box [519201]
Sharjah, UAE
www.austinmacauley.ae
+971 655 95 202

Table of Contents

Foreword

I have struggled with anxiety since I was twelve years old. Over five decades, I wrestled with this unwieldy foe. I have felt it in a house full of people. I have felt it at the end of a busy day, after I've done everything I'm supposed to do. I have felt it driving to the grocery store. It has sat with me in church. It has joined me while at a table seated with family for Thanksgiving dinner. I have stepped off airplanes in some of the most interesting cities in the world, and it has been waiting for me. I have finished speaking – sharing intimate details about my life – and it has wrapped itself around my heart and mind. I have had a great day when something amazing has happened, and it's still there. I have had a hard day, facing painful realities, and it is my constant companion. I have willed it to go away, and it returns, proving it is stronger than my will. I have tried to numb myself to it with food, alcohol, shopping, work, or people-pleasing – only to find that it is actually strengthened by these attempts to escape. I have prayed for it to go away and it becomes part of my prayer.

I picked up Jason Sullivan's book, *Quiet Chaos,* with a great deal of ambivalence. Many people don't understand anxiety – either dismissing it as trivial or stigmatizing it as something not human. I wondered what Jason would have to say about this tricky topic. I was not disappointed. Jason understands anxiety. He bravely throws his story into the mix with the rest of us who struggle with desire gone haywire. He does not shirk back from telling the truth about the dark and desperate places anxiety can take us. He is one of us.

Jason does not stop by simply empathizing with those of us who know anxiety. He digs deeper to help us know anxiety in new ways – in ways that are transformative. He explains the origins of anxiety, the brain chemistry of anxiety, and all the symptoms of anxiety. I read my story in his words and breathed a sigh of relief, *"He gets it."*

Jason's book is not just filled with information. This tale of transformation tells the truth about anxiety but does not leave us there. As I read further in this book, I thought of the words of psychoanalyst Carl G. Jung, *"What you resist persists."* This book compellingly examines anxiety so that we don't have to hide it in the basement of our lives. We can stop resisting the shame of it and start breathing in peace.

Chinese philosopher Lao Tzu wrote, *"The greatest gift you have to give is that of your own self-transformation."* Jason's compassionate understanding of anxiety invites us to engage our minds and our hearts to allow anxiety to metamorphize into a new reality. Anxiety can be a weight consuming our strength. As you read this book, you will find yourself starting to hope that shedding the weight is possible. Moving forward from anxiety is possible. Much like the butterfly wrestling through the layers of its cocoon, you will dare to believe that you don't have to be weighed down by anxiety. You are meant to use your wings.

Anxiety keeps us from accepting who we really are. This beautiful book of information and transformation heralds the oh-too-good-to-be-true news: anxiety is not a bad ending. It can be a beginning to something good. Once again, from the wisdom of Lao Tzu, *"What the caterpillar calls the end, the rest of the world calls a butterfly."*

Jason, thank you for this beautiful, strong book. Thank you for giving us a resource to see our strengths more clearly than we can by ourselves. Your words pull us into hope and freedom.

Sharon A. Hersh, M.A., LPC
Sharon is a licensed professional counselor, author, professor, and speaker. She teaches graduate counseling classes in Addiction and Sexuality and speaks at conferences and retreats. She wrote the best-selling *Bravehearts: Unlocking the Courage to Love with Abandon* as well as the acclaimed *The Last Addiction: Why Self-Help is Not Enough.* Her new book, *Belonging: Finding The Way Back to One Another* will be released in 2020. Sharon lives in Lone Tree, Colorado.

Part I

Perception and Awareness

"If the doors of perception were cleansed, everything would appear to man as it is, infinite."

— William Blake, *The Marriage of Heaven and Hell.*

Chapter 1
Throw Me a Rope

I am a man of failures. I can sabotage a moment, a person, myself, before I even know it has happened. I never intend to; in fact, my intentions tend, at least for the most part, to be good. I love people, I want to see the best for those around me, and then my heart breaks because I have done it once again. I remember as a child, fearing that God hated me, not for any specific reason, just for the simple fact that I was.

Growing up in an abusive home was no help. The moments of fear that gripped me, stayed with me, paralyzed my heart, and reinforced so many of the thoughts that, to this day, haunt my soul. Words are powerful. They can build, destroy, forgive, and even break us without being spoken. We think in words, and those words are carried from other times, both good and bad. They serve as markers, ways that we define and understand ourselves, as well as others. My markers, for the most part, have never been good. There have been positive words, of course, but for some reason, I don't like them. I am afraid to cling to them. I question them. What if they are wrong? Would that make me naïve to some central fault in myself? I don't want to overlook my weaknesses; I want to be aware of them because after all, I am destructive. I have seen the work of my faults, and they have hurt a lot of people. I have seen the work of other's faults too, and left unchecked; they destroyed the heart of a young man who wanted only to be loved. They caused countless volumes of second thoughts, regrets, and regrets of decisions made on those regrets. I seamlessly constructed a world where I was, by default, the protagonist, and the world had to painstakingly endure my existence.

As a therapist, I meet daily with many who are skilled in these arts. I want to leap from my chair and give them the lens from which I view them. I want to dry their tears and show them the difference between who they see and who they truly are, and then after those moments, I descend from wanting to liberate the captive hearts merely to return to my own captivity.

This is not the typical book on 'self-help.' I cannot offer sunshine and green meadows for the heart. Rather, I am offering something else, something that many books omit; honesty. I am inviting the reader to walk a short while with me into a greater depth. I cannot, with any good conscience, offer you simple answers, for if these were simple questions, they would have been resolved without the need for any help.

One of the many problems that we face on a daily basis is that of expectations. We are bombarded from every direction. Marketing alone questions our masculinity, femininity, competence, and general state of being as a defined goal of introducing to us a product or solution which will offer resolve. We face expectations from our cultures, societal norms, families, friends, and none of them seem to agree on any fact, other than we do not accomplish them well.

A dear friend of mine passed away recently. He was a very polarizing person. Many made judgments of him based on his actions, which in all honesty, were constantly in conflict. He was a man of extremes. He wanted to know love and would work to be a desirable person. His understanding of being desirable meant doing good things and looking the part. He would focus on his faith and would endure endless self-afflicted abuse. After months of pain, isolation, and loneliness, he would abandon his conservative ground and flee to passion and his self-defined hedonism. We had many deep conversations about life, desire, friendship, but they would be followed by deep sabotage. He would vanish from the landscape of our friendship only to reappear weeks, sometimes months, later torn, broken, and bleeding (sometimes literally), with tear-filled eyes. His honesty, in those moments, would shame the most religious man's confessions. His problem was not that he wasn't aware of his struggles, it was not that he lacked in conviction, it was that he was in conflict with who he was and who he thought he should be. I find that to be a common issue. Who are we? Who am I?

Solving the Problem that doesn't exist

It doesn't matter who you are, how confident you may be, there is a side of yourself that you are hiding. I am not exempt from this either. There is a darker side to us, a dark space that we omit from the outside world. It is this separation, this sense of shame that causes such deep conflict. The more we work to hide the darkness in us, the greater the intensity of conflict emerges and mostly, will end in some form of sabotage.

Isolation becomes a solution that engulfs the darkness and eventually our entirety. We are taught from very young ages, to perform and be seen as something more than we are. It is often given in simple answers. When we water down a complex problem with simple solutions and numb ourselves to the reality that these are not answers, we become increasingly numb to the fact that we have created a problem that didn't exist.

To test this idea is very simple; ask a child. Children have not learned or at least, honed the skill of hiding from realities. They will simply tell you, not processing any scenarios or padding any truths. They have not learned to hide the simple facts, they possess an honesty that most of us have lost as we have aged.

The Problem of Truth

Life is an unfoldment, and the further we travel, the more truth we can comprehend. To understand the things that are at our door is the best preparation for understanding those that lie beyond.

Hypatia had more reasons for avoiding self-understanding and truth than many of us do and yet, she penned such powerful words.

The problem of truth is that it requires us to examine what is at our door. Most of us like the idea of truth just as we like the idea of love, marriage, and work, however, the active pursuit and the reality of it are often terrifying. It means that we must face what is standing in the quiet, dark regions in our own lives, the deep and buried secrets which were carefully tucked away, along with the honesty to accept that it is ultimately part of what makes us who we are.

Therapists will often use terms like living an 'authentic life' or 'being real' when it comes to consciously living in the tension between our inner shame and the outside world. While this may be true, it still compartmentalizes the idea. It still suggests that an authentic life is truly authentic or that being real is constantly real. Even these terms can become an escape from the grasp of truth. It provides a sense of achievement that has a beginning and is manageable. The problem, simply put, is that truth is not manageable. It can threaten our sense of security in any situation, and this is, in very real terms, a nightmare that we live with on a daily basis.

Until you make the unconscious conscious, it will direct your life, and you will call it fate.
The pendulum of the mind oscillates between sense and nonsense, not between right and wrong.
One does not become enlightened by imagining figures of light, but by making the darkness conscious.

Jung pulls us further down the path of darkness stating that, by default, we avoid these unconscious truths to the point that the truth that we deny the most, exerts the most power over us. We become, in effect, a slave to our shame and thus, through our denial and avoidance, we bring the truth to light.

This is a problematic issue as our avoidance is a mechanism to detach from that truth. Therefore, we create cycles and patterns each more complex than the last, more disconnected from the primary cause and hence, closer to nonsense. This, in turn, pushes us away from the norms that we covet. Eventually, we become detached enough from these norms, this is called a disorder. Not all disorders are environmentally based, but all are directly impacted by our stance and coping strategies around more profound truths.

We are hardwired to be social creatures. It is in our D.N.A. This is true, even to the point that we will isolate traits in ourselves which are not seen as savory or acceptable in our social worlds. This inevitably has a spiral effect, in that the harder we work to isolate traits, the more of ourselves we isolate and eventually, we lose our social connections due to fear, shame, and avoidance. This has a paralytic effect on our lives. We often become convinced that we hide things because we are aware of them, and that common sense would dictate that the implications that these truths would have more significant effects if they were known by others. I would posit that we hide them because we want to be unaware and that we hunger for a level of intimacy that could embrace them. We are, in turn, so terrified that rather than intimacy, we face rejection, rejection compounded with the fact that we are rejected as we are, not as we want to be seen. We would be in a condition of helplessness left to drift down a river of lonely despair, isolated because that fear, the fear that we are more than anyone could handle, was confirmed. Yes, we would be drifting alone with no one to throw us a rope, no one to console us, as we experience such a dark night of the soul. This is the sabotage that we work so well. We are not choosing to hide truths to make us more socially acceptable. We are choosing to drift down a river of despair on our own terms. We are attempting to rewire the D.N.A. of a socially developed creature who is afraid of failing. Failing and confirming that there was never any control of the truths which threatened to undo us. It is a losing battle, and therefore, we program our minds to determine our value based on the lowest common denominator. Outwardly, we look successful and social, but inwardly, we base our value in the deep labyrinth of darkness that dwells below the surface of our existence, that which we have waged a lifelong war to hide. This is the cycle of shame.

How do we overcome this war, this cycle of isolation? Can we? The path of this journey is winding and most of the time, counter-intuitive. There are no simple answers; the comfort we gained from black and white categories is exchanged for gray and shades of grays. Our system of managing truth and navigating isolation will fall swiftly by the wayside with every step. This means that finding true comfort and security will mean letting go the old vices which gave us a manufactured sense of control and rest.

When we begin to embrace not only truth, but the reality of being seen as we truly are, we will find ourselves in uncharted territory. Truth can be an overwhelming foe or an irrepressible ally. Neither may offer an answer that we want to embrace, but if we understand more clearly our place in the process, it may not matter. What if the answer isn't to be more, to be better, to work harder, and to keep a stiff upper lip? What if we didn't have to have it all together and what if that was okay? Yes, it would mean great risk; it would threaten the gauge of self-importance, but what if we were not as important as we thought we were? What if the challenge was not about proving to the world and ourselves that we are enough? Maybe the process is so tough and daunting because we are learning more about being than doing. Being, this word just doesn't have the same impact as doing. No one ever calls you and says, 'How are you being?' They want to know what you are doing! We are given evaluations, throughout life, to tell us that we are doing the right things the right ways. It could be an exam, a yearly evaluation of your work performance, but it seems like the same question, what are you doing! Have you ever taken an evaluation that was based on your state of being as opposed to the amount of effort that was put into providing the expected answers? We live in a society, in a world, that is very interested in your ability to achieve and how to quantify that ability into worth. When you first meet someone, one of the first questions that is asked is usually, 'What do you do for a living?' Why does this take precedence over who is the substance of you? The sad reality is that for many, what you do is an equivalency to who you are. This is not to say that simply because someone asks what you do for a living, that it is an assumption that they do not want to know who you are. Rather, the fact is that it has become such a normal equivalency that very few notice or question it. The answer to the question functions the same way. We usually say, 'I am a doctor, lawyer, builder…' Even our processing of the question is to assume that what I do is who I am. I believe we may be putting the cart before the horse. You are far less than you fear you are, and much more than you communicate. Understanding that, is an act of balance and honesty that challenges each of us to the core. I put this course of thinking to the test a few years ago. Someone whom I had met asked me, "So, Jason, what do you do for a living?" My response was, "Well, I mess up a lot, I apologize, try to see things from other's perspectives, gain a little more knowledge of myself, and separate the fact that when I make a mistake, that it does not define me as a bad person, just a person that makes mistakes. I do that and repeat it a lot." There was an awkward pause. I could see that this was much more than was expected in the answer. I let the awkwardness hang in the air for a moment and then said, "But I get paid to do therapy." There was a look of relief and a chuckle from both sides.

Before we can begin to understand who we are, who we truly are, we have to stop muddying the waters by trying to prove who we want to think we are. This goes against many schools of thought present in today's world. Some would say that we are only as important as we think we are, others would say that what you do is who you are, and yet, others would tell you that the universe is at your beck and call, waiting in hopes that you will embrace your inner destiny, take the reins, and become its co-conspirator. I will address these ideas more fully later, but for now, let us assume only this, you are not as important as you fear you are, and you are much more than you communicate (whether you are a narcissist or not).

There are so many ways that I fear not being good enough. I question myself on a daily basis. I ache to receive affirmation, and when I receive it, I take it, tear it apart, and find ways to dismiss it. I am afraid of becoming complacent and yet, in my fear of complacency, I drink from a stagnated pool of criticisms assuming that if it is negative, it must be true. This is a reflection of how I see myself, and I don't have room for sunshine, roses, and kittens. I can take the negative because in some ways, I'm relieved that the negative isn't quite as bad as I see myself. That means they haven't figured me out yet.

The positive, I file away in one of the following categories: stuff you're supposed to say to be nice, flattery, and stuff you think you know about me, but don't really know, because there's an entirely different side of me that never sees the light of the day, and if you knew that side of me, you would grab your things and run for the door.

The last category is a bit lengthy, but it is quite full.

So what does it mean to grow? There are approaches, gimmicks, strategies, and five-step plans that can keep you running and striving for an idealized existence. Many of these are founded with good intentions, and for some, they act as a salve to soothe the aching heart. What if there was more than good intention and an appearance of wholeness? What if growth was less about constructing a better you? It seems that in the many approaches and theories that exist, they share one common assertion, and that is that something is missing in each of us. Otherwise, I would not be looking for steps or solutions. The fault with most of these approaches is that they assert a linear approach to growth. I would assert that growth is not linear and thus, there will be much confusion and frustration surrounding any approach that embraces such a foundational concept.

We do not grow absolutely, chronologically. We grow, sometimes in one dimension, and not in another; unevenly.

We grow partially. We are relative. We are mature in one realm, childish in another. The past, present, and future mingle and pull us backward, forward, or fix us in the present. We are made up of layers, cells, constellations.

Anais Nin gives us some insight into the complexity of identity and growth. In short, we are all complicated messes. We know it, and we hate it. We feel shame, sadness, fear, and disappointment. These are vulnerable emotions, and thus, in the complexity of our brains, we create coping strategies to help us survive the fear of being discovered as incompetent, weak, insecure, and lonely, or just bad. The root desire is to be loved, known and loved, but our fear tells us that there is something uniquely wrong with us; wrongness that is so different, so ugly, that if the world knew it, they would surely reject us and we would be left known and unloved. Our coping strategies attempt to offer a compromise. This compromise is to be unknown and loved to the depth that we can be transparent.

It is as if the entire world has thrown a masquerade party and each person designs the mask that will present the ideal 'them.' When the guests arrive, they are so ornately disguised that we become enamored with the masks. The more we notice and compliment the covering, the more we treat it as if it was the reality of the person. Over time, resentment builds over the divide between the mask and what lies beneath. We despise the fact that the world loves the mask and yet, doesn't know the one concealed by its elegant beauty.

I find that, in every relationship, you are engaging with two people. One is the person that you hope that they are, and the other is the person that they truly are. This compounds the issue of transparency. The person that we hope someone is: a set of expectations and assumptions. This means that we are looking into the mask and adding our own decorations. We may idealize the person, or even underestimate them. They see us through the same dualistic way. Do we embrace the mask with all its adornment, or the scarred and insecure person beneath?

21

My tendency is to assume the best. I reach out to the mask and admire its intricacy. I am often enamored by the shine and splendor of what lies before me. This leads me down a long and winding road. Left with these assumptions, I am forced to introspect on the flaws that lie beneath my own mask. If this person is this well put together, if they are this amazing, I am even more of a disaster than I realized. In my idealization of the mask, I ultimately emphasize my own insecurity. This is not a pedestal to which I elevate another. Rather, it is a deep pit in which I dig myself into a trench of isolation and fear; a fear of being exposed as a fake, a fraud, and once exposed being known and rejected. Reject my mask, please reject the mask, but don't reject the broken man behind it. This is the cry of many hearts and the paralyzing reality in which many of us live.

The second pitfall that this assumption creates is disappointment. I have disappointed many people and disappointed them deeply. I have failed their expectations, and upon removing my own mask, I have been left lonely, broken, and bleeding. I have been called a saint and sinner by the same person, I have been told that they would never throw their pearls in front of me, insinuating that I am literally a swine, unworthy of their time or attention. I remember the feelings that ensued shortly after these conversations; anger, mixed exquisitely with fear, sadness, and hopelessness. I never claimed to be whole; I never, knowingly, laid out an image of myself that was intended to be so far from the reality of the real me. Yet, based on the assumptions that I failed, the deep contrast between the mask and the man beneath it, I was truly known and painfully rejected. I isolated myself to new depths. I cut myself from everyone I knew, wholly out of the fear that I would be exposed further. I hated myself, probably more than the person in front of me. I could not undo the exposure, the disappointment; I could only crawl away with the affirmation that I was much worse than I thought I was, and slip back to my dark cave of isolation and false comfort.

This caused waves of grief and constant sabotage. I lost my friends, eventually my spouse. I threw myself into the only safe place I could find, and that was work. I excelled as a therapist and found a new mask. After my divorce, I plummeted even deeper. I was truly alone. I had a couple of friends that were there for me, no matter what. They were the lifeline that I couldn't break. They knew me, they loved me, and when I would pull out the mask to cover my shame, they would patiently and carefully remove it for it was the scarred and broken person beneath that they truly loved. I did rebel. I broke just about every moral constraint that I had. I assumed the worst of myself and I was driven to find the bottom. Over the next two years, I would make discoveries of myself and the horrid mistakes that, to this day, haunt me.

One of these mistakes came out of a carnal curiosity. I remember it clearly. I was on holiday, driving fifteen or so hours. As I drove, billboards began to appear; Adult entertainment, strippers, fully nude. Each billboard piqued my desire for escape and curiosity. I had never visited a strip club. I had been staunchly opposed to them. I saw them as meat markets for unrestrained cannibals. That night, that moment, I was the cannibal. I pulled into the parking lot. I walked into the club expecting something that would numb the previous hours of quietly violent, self-asserted abuse. I ordered a drink and sat down. There were several men there. Each looked lonelier than the last, each existing at that moment, in a sort of daze. I was no exception. There were the regulars, those who had become so accustomed to the numbness that they had developed an air of confidence. One man referred to one of the ladies by name and uttered a series of expletives that were demeaning and showed the utter depth of separation between the man who he was and the identity that he had forged.

After several minutes of sitting, watching, a lady approached me. She took my hand and led me to a backroom. She began to dance seductively. She removed one piece of what little clothing covered her. It was at this moment that the dam of reality broke. I looked into her eyes and what I saw was not a seductive woman bent on enticing me. I saw a deep emptiness, a sense of sadness that can only be described as hopelessness. This time, I took her hand, "Wait. Please, stop.

23

Sit down. I don't want to be another person that pushes you down this road. Tell me about yourself." Her expression was that of shock, almost fear. Maybe she was afraid of being seen in a different type of exposure. Maybe she thought I was a serial killer. Regardless, she sat innocently beside me. She told me her real name. She told me that she had a son and that the father of this son had left. She hadn't finished high school, she dropped out to work and support her boy. She began to weep. She wept deeply. She said some of the most powerful words that I had heard in a long time, "I hate this; I hate being this person that dances while men stare. I'm shy, I hate this life, but what else can I do? If I don't work, my son doesn't eat, doesn't have a home. I want him to have all the things that I never did, and if it means that I have to be this, this object, then it is worth it, I guess." It had gone from an awkwardly attempted lap dance to a real conversation. We were both in tears. As she described her life, more of how she saw her role in it, the way that she had been objectified, and even abused, I realized that upon entering the club, I was just another man looking for an escape at the cost of someone else's dignity. I apologized for being the very thing that she described. As we walked back from the room, I left a part of myself there. At the most profound moment of despair, I began to understand that even though I had acted on my own selfish desires that it was not who I was. It was a portion, a part of a greater whole. It was a messy part of a messier whole, but it served as a wake-up call. How many times had I furthered my own agenda of self-gratification at the expense of someone else? Maybe it wasn't in a strip club, perhaps it was a sarcastic comment that momentarily elevated my status in some social setting, and perhaps it was pulling on the exposed weakness of a vulnerable and honest person. However I looked at it, I was guilty, guilty and exposed more deeply than any stripper had ever been. I began to realize that my mechanism of assumed confidence was only a fragile shell that served to protect me from a real world with real hurt. That night in a strip club, I found that I was the predator looking to devour something, someone more vulnerable than I was willing or honestly aware enough to be. I never returned to another club; I never went back to devour, stare, or feed my now-broken mask. I realized that there are two types of people when it comes to removing their masks. There are those that choose to remove it in an act of bravery, staunchly poised to reveal themselves in a moment that could serve to be more costly if the face behind it is rejected. Then there are those, the group that I fit into, those that have their mask torn away. They are exposed, they have nothing left to lose, and no one left to lose. This is not about bravery, but more directly desperation. As I sat, more exposed than I ever intended, I chose to do it differently. A choice that has moved me forward as a person, has caused me pain on many levels, but has left me with a confidence that allows me to experience moments without my mask.

Chapter 2
Wherever the Road Leads

It was in March of 2010 that I made a life-changing decision. Before I go further, it is important to understand my love for my home. My heart will always be in Florida. My dream to return stays with me, but now is not the time. 2009 was a disastrous year. I watched my private practice grow. I was excelling, and by this point, I was working out of two offices, with a client base of around sixty plus. I was working six-day weeks. I was engrossed in improving and growing this practice into something more. I was enamored with success and feeding the emptiness within myself that lied just beneath the surface. While I was a successful therapist, I was a terrible husband. I had it all figured out in my head. I told myself and the world around me that I wanted to establish my career so that I could provide a stable home that would allow my future children to flourish. The saddest portion was that I was probably the only one that believed it. My marriage was withering. I was neglecting my role as a husband in the name of providing, while in reality, not only was I not providing, I was abandoning my role. My pride/bottomless pit of fear that I may not be enough engulfed me and ultimately ruined a marriage. I was toxic and had intoxicated my marriage. I gave my spouse every reason to leave. By the time I realized it, it was too late. The damage which could not be undone had been done. Though I had lost my marriage and even understood my faults, I saw myself as a victim of circumstance. This was not a simple story nor can I tell it with objectivity. All that I can say is that I starved a marriage to the point of death. I still had my practice, and I dove more deeply than ever into it. The more I worked, the more my business grew. I became a member of the Florida Crisis Response Team. I responded to disasters and excelled there as well. I had an affinity for distancing myself from the emotion of calamity which served well at a disaster site. Unfortunately, this does not fare well in life. You can visit a disaster, you can make a difference, but you can't live there.

A friend of mine invited me to work in Bahrain, to set up a practice. I was good with marketing and therapy, and they saw this as a good fit. After a lot of discussion, and ignorance on my part, I spoke with another friend who was working in Kuwait. I wanted to know what life in the region was like. I had a very limited concept of the Middle East. It was constrained to C.N.N. and Call of Duty. Much to my surprise, my inquisitive call turned into a job offer. There was an opening at a university in Kuwait. "You should apply! Why would you start over in practice when you could step into a stable job with a contract?" I politely refused and returned to my inquisitive tone. After the conversation, I sat with two men who I deeply trust. These are men who have seen the worst sides of me and have stood by me. They are much further down the road of wisdom than I could ever dream of being, and I value their input and friendship more than I can ever communicate. I mentioned the offer to them. Both asked why I would leave an established practice to move to something unknown. I agreed. After all, I had tied my identity so much to my job that I would not only be leaving my practice, but as much of myself as I knew at the time. As time passed, I worked long hours and slept very little. When there was no work, I had to face the abysmal truth of my own existence, so I filled that time with nightclubs, alcohol, parties, friends, hobbies, and anything else that would allow me avoid the enormous hole in my chest. Over time, it began to take its toll on me. I was always tired, always moving from one thing to another, one relationship after another. I didn't even know what I was looking for anymore. I just knew that if I stopped for even for a moment, my entire world would fall apart. I didn't want to be known and loved; I didn't want to be known at all. I was like a shadow floating from one place to the next. No substance, no presence, just an absence of light surviving in darkness.

I believe that we idealize isolation. Relationships are complicated and consume so much of us. They require us to be honest, honest with those around us, and honest with ourselves. I was not having any part of that. When we isolate, we can dream of what it would be like to find that one person, the one person that would complete us, understand us. We have an innate desire to be exposed fully and loved, in spite of our faults. What a beautiful dream! As long as we maintain our isolation, it is a safe and beautiful dream. We can eliminate the awkwardness of learning to risk and trust. We can control every aspect of the person we conceive in our minds, and once again, we fall in love with another mask. This is a mask of our own making which accompanies a lonely heart. It is romantic, soft, tender, but much like all the other devices of isolation, it is empty. If we are looking for someone to complete us, we are placing an expectation on someone else to do the work of honesty, intimacy, and worst of all risk.

As the time passed, the subject of Kuwait came up again, "Jason, what is going on with the Kuwait offer?"

"Nothing really, it was an offer, and I said no."

"Maybe you should consider it. You have not been yourself in a long time. You have drifted, something big is missing in you." Something about that conversation had a tremendous impact on me. It made me consider this truly foreign idea. That night, I sat down with my laptop and sent an email that would go on to change everything I had ever known.

"Is the job offer still available? I've been thinking that maybe a change would be good for me." The next day, I received a reply, "Yes! Can you interview today? We need to fill the position this week." We set a time for the interview, and in one call, I was bound for a new world. It was now May of 2010, and my starting date was August 1st. The next few months seemed like a whirlwind. At times, it felt like the ultimate escape; a new place, a new identity, a new start, but inevitably, the same me.

I remember stepping on to the plane, tears in my eyes, as I was leaving the place that I called home. I was leaving my friends, my life behind for what? An unknown existence, and a country that I was only aware of because of two wars? My mind raced during the flight; I vacillated between thoughts of a new experience and the world that I was leaving behind.

Twenty-two hours later, I landed in Kuwait. I was greeted by my friend at the airport. I didn't feel like I was in a different country, I felt like I was on a different planet. The following weeks, I realized how easy it was to isolate myself. My phone was silent, I didn't know where anything was, and I existed in one of two places; home and work. I got exactly what I had wanted. I was alone and on my own, away from a world of trouble, alone, alone.

It took time to meet friends and often, I would avoid meeting outside of work. I have an anxiety disorder; a disorder that has haunted me since childhood. A disorder that I was not aware of until it was out of control. I was diagnosed in 2004. I was working on my master's degree. I was eager to learn but was such a terrible student. The irony of being a person who loves to learn but does not excel in a classroom was unfathomable to most of my teachers, professors, and my parents. I couldn't focus, I would forget things constantly. Nights before exams, I would sit, staring at books and notes unable to read, paralyzed by worry. I thought it was both, normal and that I just was lazy or I was not as smart as I should be.

The first time it became an issue was in second grade. My mother received a phone call, "Hello, this is Mrs. Rogers, Jason's teacher. We are very concerned about Jason. We think that he may have some issues, he may be retarded." This was the first school-related beating that I had ever received. "What is wrong with you? They think you are retarded! They want to test you! What are you doing in school that would make anyone think such things?" Within days, I was given an assessment. The results led to my second school-related beating. "So, you're not retarded! They say you're 'gifted.' They want to promote you to the next grade. I told them that he doesn't deserve to be promoted to anything; he is just lazy and I will deal with that!" I remember the pain of the belt as it struck my legs, my shoulders, my back, my chest, and eventually, my face. The assessment showed that rather than the expected lower I.Q., I had a higher I.Q. than average. I still question the validity of that assessment. Most parents would be relieved, maybe even excited, to find that their child was smarter than they thought, but my family was different. There was only lazy. No one wanted to be inconvenienced with calls from the school over concerns of my performance. It was frustrating, it was a bother, and there were more important things to deal with than my laziness. I can say that there was more attention given to my performance, not necessarily the helpful kind. The new rule was failing expectations means punishment. There were many failures and a lot of punishment. I did survive second grade, but what was engrained in my mind now was not just anxiety, but deep fear. Fear of failure and all that it entailed.

When I entered the third grade, I learned a new trick, silence. I remember that in December of that year, I gave up. I literally just stopped speaking. I didn't say a word for months, and no one noticed. I wasn't beaten; there was no yelling; it was peaceful. No one noticed. Except for one person, Mrs. Huff, my teacher. This, of course, signaled another phone call, "Hello, this is Mrs. Huff, Jason's teacher. We are a bit concerned. Jason is doing well with his work, but he just doesn't speak. He doesn't have friends. He just does his work and nothing more. We are concerned that he may not be socially ready for the fourth grade." My mother was not pleased, to say the least, "Again!? I am being called into the school not because you are retarded, but because you don't have friends? What is wrong with you? Why can't you just be a normal child?" I had developed, what I would later discover is called Selective Mutism. What a great disorder! I could be invisible, I could have my thoughts to myself, and the best part was, no beatings! That all ended with the phone call. My mother screamed and beat me for what seemed to be hours. It came in waves. Yelling, hitting, leaving the room, coming back, yelling, beating, leaving, and it continued for quite some time. There was a meeting scheduled to discuss my academic fate. The teacher was encouraging. Maybe she sensed that there was much more under the surface, maybe she was just a kind person. My mother was having none of it. The ride home was long, full of yelling and words that cut deeply into a young heart. That night, I was beaten until I spoke. My first words in months, "Please, stop, I'm sorry for being bad, I'm sorry, please, stop!" As the years moved forward, it became an expectation that I would be odd, 'weird,' and 'in my own world.' It was as if my mother had given up on the hopes that I would ever be any more than just a problem. My grades remained the same; I was a solid C student. This followed me through high school, college, and eventually culminated into a breakdown during my masters. I just couldn't do it anymore. It was too much.

I walked into the dean's office and apologized like a child waiting to be beaten, "Dr. Mawhinney, I'm sorry, but I don't think that I belong here. I had three finals today, and I missed all of them. I have six papers that were due weeks ago, and I haven't even begun them. I think that I am just not that smart."

"Jason, have a seat." It was then that this kind and gentle man reached for his computer. He looked at my schedule and sighed, "Jason, no wonder you are falling apart! You took seventeen hours, and all are very demanding classes. Jason, the fact that you are here means that you are smart enough, I think that there is more to this. I will speak with your professors, and you will have extra time to complete your work. Will you do two things for me? Go home, rest, sleep, and secondly, would you meet with a counselor? I think it would help you." I literally cried in his office. I went in expecting to be berated, rejected, and instead, I was embraced, cared for, and helped.

I did follow through on my end of the deal. I met with a therapist. It took about two sessions to determine that I had severe anxiety and panic attacks. I didn't even know what a panic attack was! I thought that my entire existence was the same as anyone else's, and that I just was too stupid to pull it together.

That same year, we experienced four hurricanes. The odds of one hurricane are not that low but four, four was unheard of. The first hurricane was more like a party. We huddled in one house, all the neighbors joined. We ate, drank; we went out into the storm. As devastating as these storms are, they can be fun. After the first storm passed, I drove around the city to see the damage. As I was driving, I felt dizzy, lightheaded; I felt my heart rate increase, I began to feel pain in my chest, I thought I was dying. I stopped the car because I thought I was going to pass out. I sat for several minutes, waiting for the end to come. About fifteen minutes later, I felt better, but the worry, the worry stayed. I didn't like that feeling; I didn't want it to happen again. I told my therapist about it in our next session. He told me that it was a severe panic attack.

I was amazed, "These things have levels?"

He laughed and said, "Yes, you had a severe panic attack." As we worked more on my past and present, things took a turn for the worse. My panic attacks increased, and I began to experience sleep paralysis. Again, I brought this to my session. My therapist encouraged me to visit a doctor and begin medication for my anxiety disorder.

I was completely shocked, "Am I that crazy that I need meds? I exercise, I am a vegetarian, and I am healthy! Why would I need meds?" The reality was that I was in denial. Later that week, I had sleep paralysis again. This time, it was worse. I couldn't breathe, I couldn't move, I was utterly terrified! The next morning, I called the doctor.

The receptionist answered, "Good morning, how may I help you?"

"Yes, I need to see the doctor. My therapist says that I need to begin medication for anxiety and I agree."

"Well, let me see, we can fit you in two weeks from now. Would that work?"

"Nooooo... Two weeks from now would not 'work' for me. I have panic attacks, I'm afraid I'm dying, and I wake up unable to move or breathe. So, no, two weeks will not work at all."

"Oh, dear, that's terrible! Please, come now." Where was all of this kind mercy coming from? A dean that takes a failing student under his care, a therapist that stuck with me, and now, a receptionist that actually bumped me from two weeks to now? I was so confused; I was used to being written off as a failure and as someone for whom there was little hope. Regardless, I ran to my car, drove to the doctor's office, and for lack of a better term, I vomited all of my fear and experiences to her.

"Jason, you're not crazy! This is very common. I see so many of these cases. The medication will help, but the therapy will definitely be beneficial. Stay with it; you will be fine."

Within four weeks, I felt strangely normal. I could concentrate, I could function. I pulled out my surfboard for the first time in months, and surfed! The best part, no panic attacks! I continued therapy with a renewed fervor. We tackled issues; we talked about the years of abuse, the dysfunction of a family of addicts, the power of words, and the journey of overcoming years and years of damage. I fell in love with the process. I read every book I could get my hands on, I listened to lectures online, and then it dawned on me... This is what I want to do.

My next counseling session came. I sat down and with every ounce of conviction in me, I asked, "Am I too messed up to be a therapist?" My therapist laughed and with his kind and gentle manner, looked at me, really looked at me, and said, "Jason, you will be an excellent therapist."

Later that week, I applied to change my major to Mental-Health Counseling. I was accepted. Not just into the program, I was accepted by my therapist, my doctor, my dean, and even the kind receptionist who had every right to make me wait out two weeks, but had the kindness of heart to make room for me that day.

I have lived with Generalized Anxiety Disorder since childhood. I still find it hard, at times, to deal with life; intimacy still terrifies me. I have made more mistakes than I can count and with years of work, I can finally say that I'm not a total failure. I still have a lot of work to do, and there are so many days that I just don't like myself. There are days where the cutting words of an abusive parent still ring in my ears. I still tear up when I think of the mercy that I experienced in those years. I want to be that kind of person. I want to be the mercy that people can experience, the kind of mercy that is tangible, that has substance, and is unwavering in its resolve. I am still two people; the major difference is that I am aware.

I have lived in Kuwait for eight years. During my first year, I flew home to visit my friends and family. I got to spend time with my friend, Dan. Dan is one of the honest, transparent, and loving people that you could ever find. He's funny, he's real, and he will tell you the harder truths in a way that pulls you closer to him. He is truly a genius. While we were talking, he asked me how it felt to live abroad.

I said, "Dan, it's definitely an adventure, but I am lonely. I feel desperately alone. My anxiety piques, and I shut down." Dan knows that I am an extrovert, and that being alone is terrifying to me.

He listened intently and said these few words, words that changed how I viewed loneliness: "Jason, sometimes you have to learn to enjoy your own company." I had never thought of it this way. I never thought of being my own company. It seems so obvious, but for me, it was an elusive truth that I probably had subconsciously avoided for years. My own company? Me? I'm the last person in the world that I would want to spend time with, and yet, there I was, living in a new country, spending massive amounts of time with myself… Yay! I was not at all happy about this concept, but nonetheless, I trust my friend. He is wise beyond his years, and if he is telling me that I need to learn to enjoy my own company then damn it, I'm going to learn to enjoy my own company. As the trip home came to an end, I was faced once again with the dry thoughts of loneliness and the underwhelming idea of 'enjoying my own company.' I spent the next two years with these words on repeat. Strangely enough, some things began to change. Now don't get too excited, yes, it was an epiphany, and if the journey ended here, there would be no need to write a book. Things changed, and like many questions in life, as we look for answers, we are introduced to fewer answers and more questions.

This is indeed where I found myself. I had new categories for life, more receptacles to make sense of the world around me, and more questions begging to be answered. Somehow, there was a sense of comfort in this. I began to travel, alone. I started to explore new hobbies, alone. The irony is that as you find comfort in your own company and as you begin to explore those inner recesses concealed within your being, you also begin to move. You do explore your interests, and along the way, you find yourself surrounded with people who have similar interests, similar fears, and eventually, you call them friends.

Chapter 3
No Simple Answers

If you are suffering from panic and severe anxiety, you are not alone. According to the World Health Organization, there are 264 million documented cases in the world. These are only the documented cases. Taking into account the worldwide variations of accessibility to mental health treatment, avoidance of treatment, and diagnosis, the number is most assuredly higher.

Over the years, I have treated hundreds of cases dealing with anxiety disorders. As a matter of fact, anxiety and depression, which go hand in hand, are the most common disorders treated. When you imagine the significance of these numbers, it begs the question, "Why isn't more being done?" The reality is that there is quite a bit being done. A simple search on the web will show you page after page of answers, advertisements for treatment, medications, coloring books for anxiety, and most of these revolve around quick and simple steps. If we are left to believe the masses of information poured upon us, we find that the vast majority of it centers on a simple idea, and that is responsibility. When you go deeper into the world of mental health and anxiety, the truth is you find something dangerous; blame. Though it is often coated in kind platitudes and warm fuzzy sentiment at the root, it is blame. You have not engaged the issues you fear; you have not learned to address the issue because you avoid what you fear, your parents caused a lot of damage in your developmental years. Yes, blame, coated in the sweet therapeutic jargon of good intention. As a matter of fact, one of the most common modalities of therapy, Cognitive

Behavioral Therapy, targets simple steps, that apparently you were not smart enough to figure out on your own, and reinforces them with a presupposition that if you do it the right way long enough, you will eventually believe. In short, fake it till you make it.

Therapists pour out motivational monologues driven with the intentions of convincing you that you just don't get it. If you only work on it enough, it will all be better, and life will go on, even better than before. You will find workbooks with lists and self-assessments, book after book reminding you what a special person you are, but it's just that you can't see it because no one has allowed you to see it. I truly believe that many therapists have good intentions and are honestly misguided in their approach. Over the years, when I hire a new therapist for my department, I have asked one question, "What is your theoretical orientation?" The responses have varied from utter nonsense to yoga. I have had very few even understand the question. There is a sudden deer in the headlights look, as their mind begins to work out what that even means. It is a simple, standard question that any qualified therapist should be able to answer, but they can't! I have a wonderful staff, and I can say, in all honesty, that they are wonderful therapists, and yes, they answered the question. It is staggering to me though, that there are so many therapists who cannot even tell you what type of therapy that they practice. If a therapist has done no work in developing a clear and working model of therapy, it is time to find another therapist.

This begs the question; what type of therapy works the best? Is there a form that just works? While, in my opinion, there are better forms of therapy than others, it must also be taken into consideration that there are more personality types, than there are theories on therapy, and each person will respond differently to different types of therapy. I believe that there are tenets that we should set for a therapist, regardless of their orientation.

Setting the Bar

When I first began looking for a therapist, I asked around. I had no categories for therapy. I had no idea what I was getting myself into. I had some bad experiences and some good experiences. I was given simple answers that, just upon face value, made no logical sense. I was told by one therapist, after sharing the full unedited story of my existence, that my real issue was not anxiety. What I really needed to address was forgiveness. This led to a systemized, one-size-fits-all pamphlet about forgiving the ones that hurt us. I was told to pray and ask for forgiveness, and for the desire to forgive. Then, I was told that if I needed another session, there was an opening in six months. I was literally summed up in one session, patted on the back, and told to go pray about it. This was not therapy; it was something much worse. I left that office with one more person to forgive on an apparently long list of people to forgive. I was angry, hurt, and discouraged. Over the next several days, I began to think that something was wrong with me. Maybe I was hardened and unforgiving. Maybe I was not looking at it the right way. I questioned everything, trying to understand what I wasn't better. The therapist did tell me that if I did the work of praying and forgiving, that I would be better. I wondered if I was worse than I had communicated. Maybe there was some misunderstanding; maybe I used the wrong words. This carried me down a path of deepened anxiety and depression. He made it sound so simple and doable and yet, I couldn't do it. Now, I was not only anxious and depressed, but worried that I was going to hell, or worse, that life would work its way out to being a living hell.

So, simply put, the first rule is, there are no quick fixes or simple answers. You are not lazy; you are not unmotivated, you are anxious. You are anxious, and this is much different than lazy, in fact, it is the polar opposite of lazy, it is nonstop worry, nonstop coping, and nonstop thinking and rethinking. It is anything but lazy.

Secondly, ask upfront in the first session, "What kind of therapy do you do?" If they cannot explain it, or go into a long and unclear diatribe about growth and what it is and isn't, this is a clear sign that they don't have an answer to the question. Yes, they want to help, and yes, they may be sincere, but want and sincerity will scarcely help you with the major details of your anxiety and depression.

One of my favorite answers is that someone practices a synthetic blend of approaches. This is a common answer. My next question is, "Which practices do you blend?" If there is a pause and a blank look, then you have your answer. At this point, it is necessary to tell you that I am not pointing out one style over the other, rather that there should exist some semblance of understanding as to what it is they do.

If someone came to your office and asked you, "What do you do?" More than likely, you could rattle off a list of things that you do. If you were asked how you do it, you could more than likely explain how you do it. It's not that you are asking unreasonable questions, in fact, they are the most reasonable questions you could ask.

Thirdly, anxiety is not strictly an emotional issue. It is predominantly biological. According to the D.S.M. IV (Diagnostic and Statistical Manual, 4th edition), these are the symptoms of a panic attack:

- Palpitations, pounding heart, or accelerated heart rate.
- Sweating.
- Trembling or shaking.
- Sensations of shortness of breath or smothering.
- A feeling of choking.
- Chest pain or discomfort.
- Nausea or abdominal distress.
- Feeling dizzy, unsteady, lightheaded, or faint.
- Feelings of unreality (derealization), or being detached from oneself (depersonalization).
- Fear of losing control or going crazy.
- Fear of dying.
- Numbness or tingling sensations (paresthesia).
- Chills or hot flashes.

In that list of symptoms, how many emotional symptoms do you see? Yes, one! Fear... Fear of dying and fear of losing control. When you look at the other symptoms which all appear within a fraction of a second, I would say that fear would be a reasonable emotion to experience. It is important to find a therapist with some understanding of the brain and the body. When you begin to break down the criteria listed, you will not find a chaotic biological process where the body is on the verge of death or losing control. To the contrary, this is a very controlled and purposeful biological process. The brain is perceiving danger, imminent danger. As this danger is perceived, the limbic system, which is the first portion of the brain to process information, recognizes something that appears to be an immediate risk. This is where the brain makes a decision. Instead of sending the information to the prefrontal cortex for further processing and decision-making, it sends a signal directly to the center nervous system, telling the body to streamline its process and to send as much oxygen, sugar, and adrenaline to the arms and legs. Serotonin surges, in this case, it acts as a vascular constrictor. It is, in effect, reducing the flow of blood to the brain and rerouting it to the extremities. Now, there is more blood pushing through the heart, and the brain is prepared. It sends a signal to increase the heart rate, to push the blood more quickly to the lungs. This increase in heart rate sometimes occurs as a palpitation. The next step is oxygenating the blood. Now, a protein is released in the brain that tells the body you are suffocating. This causes a reaction which I affectionately refer to as the panic breath. It is that deep breath that you take when you feel anxious at the beginning of a panic attack. The blood is not receiving oxygen, and now it needs sugars, proteins, and carbohydrates, and another signal is sent to the digestive system. The brain is telling your stomach to produce more acid to break down food faster. This, in turn, is absorbed into the blood. Cortisol levels rise, adrenaline levels rise, body temperature fluctuates and often times, as a result of the rapid release of these hormones, there is a tingling sensation that is felt in the arms and legs. All of this... ALL OF THIS, occurs in seconds. You wonder why you feel terrified that you are going to lose control or die. I think that this is a very reasonable thought. Over time, we begin to become more and more anxious about panic attacks, we literally panic that we might panic. If a therapist can familiarize you with these steps and systems in the body, it offers the rest of your brain the opportunity to begin to normalize these symptoms. I am not saying that a therapist should be an M.D. or a psychiatrist, but it is extremely valuable to understand that there is a balance between physiology and emotion. Ask questions about your panic attack.

Fourthly, a good therapist will be a good student. He or she may have seen a thousand cases of anxiety disorders and may know the symptoms inside and out, but they have never seen your anxiety. They have never heard your story. This is important to note. You are not meeting with a psychic. We are not mind readers and should not look bored because we are hearing about another anxiety disorder. Rather, every person, every client, is an individual with a myriad of experiences that make them unique. A good therapist will listen, taking in all of the information, and learning from you. Your story is incredibly important and is worth being heard. This is the process of therapy. If you meet with a therapist and you are constantly interrupted, it can be frustrating. You need to be heard! You are on the journey of sharing the most profound and most intimate details, which are terrifying to talk about, that make you who you are. They need to be honored and treated with respect.

Finally, seven-step plans, five-steps, however many… These honestly terrify me. I know therapists that will sell you a package of five or seven sessions, assuring you that you will be all better by the time you finish. I actually get a lot of clients who come to me angry and frustrated, that they just spent $1,500 on a program/system that was supposed to cure them. I can tell you as a therapist, and as someone that suffers from Generalized Anxiety Disorder, that there are no shortcuts. People promising relief from major anxiety in a matter of weeks have either graduated from Hogwarts School of Wizardry, or they are simply just salespeople.

This should give you some basic principles in finding a therapist. There are no perfect therapists. We all make mistakes, and it is both good and ethical for us to take ownership when we make them. I will address in more detail throughout this book, various strategies and approaches that are effective in therapy. We have much more to talk about in this long process, and I will address as much as a book will allow.

Chapter 4
Panic, Sleeplessness, and Anger

Anxiety disorders vary in many ways. Some are developed through environmental stressors and trauma, while others can be hereditary. Some will last for a period of time, while others will stay with you in some form for the duration of life. They are the culmination of many systems in the body working overtime and are often accompanied by tiredness and ironically sleeplessness.

Anxiety works on a premise of control. We fear that we are, in some way, lacking the control we need to move forward, to be competent, or merely, to exist. This raises some fundamental questions. In his epilogue from the book, *Existential Psychotherapy*, Irvin Yalom has this to say:

Existential Therapy is a dynamic approach that focuses on concerns rooted in human existence. Each of us craves perdurance, groundedness, community, and pattern; and yet, we must all face inevitable death, groundlessness, isolation, and meaninglessness. Existential Therapy is based on a model of psychopathology which posits that anxiety and its maladaptive consequences are responses to these four ultimate concerns.

In essence, we are facing an existential crisis at every turn. We begin to understand that we have no control over these elements and we do not possess healthy coping strategies to rectify this reality. I believe that this is not just restricted to anxiety or an anxiety disorder. Rather, this is something that every individual must grapple with several times over the course of their life. Making this even more complex is the ever-present question of identity: Who am I?

Identity crises abound in our societies today. We have developed strata based on ideologies, wealth, social status, gender, race, fashion, and much more. This creates a group identity and group identities, while they act as an immediate solution to the identity question, ultimately undercuts individual identity. Liberal, conservative, Caucasian, Hispanic, straight, gay, lesbian, bisexual have all become terms associated with groups that individuals identify with whether in favor or not. This is, of course, a very limited list and is to be taken with the understanding that to provide a full list would exhaust volumes of books. We are desperately hungry and anxious that we may not know our identity. If we cannot even understand ourselves, it is safe to say that we cannot understand our place in the world. Therefore, we adhere ourselves to groups and ideologies that we can associate with. When we submit ourselves to a group identity, we subjugate ourselves to the rules of these ideologies, often times not contemplating the greater lengths or cost that this subjugation will require. We do not solely subscribe to one group identity either, we may find ourselves in many, and it is important to note that while there may be agreement among groups over issues or tendencies, it does not necessarily account for the totality of our being.

So, what benefits are gained from group identity? As Yalom pointed out in his epilogue; groundedness, community, and meaning play immense roles in our identity. A group ideologue offers some semblance of an answer to these questions. They give a sense of purpose, they offer a community, and within a group ideology, there is an accepted moral and intellectual structure. These are all so enticing, but do they really answer the question of who I am? I would posit that while community and shared values are important, a group ideology, on the other hand, strips the individuality from our identity. One example would be fashion. Many people spend a lot of time and money, choosing clothes and accessories deemed fashionable by a small but extremely influential minority of the population. They are not choosing clothes that express their individual perception of style but rather, choosing clothes that show that they are part of something else. We want to belong; we ache to be a part of something greater and many times, we lose the very deepest cravings of the heart at the altar of a group ideology.

We are constantly driven by affirmation through social media. How many likes did I get? How many followers do I have? These also constitute a socially agreed-upon ideology of success in social media, to the point that many live more in the world of selfies and immediate gratification through hearts and thumbs up. It is a means of connecting without connecting. It is a way of establishing a sense of, but it is also a place where much anxiety rests. Cyberbullying, trolling, hacking accounts constantly put that gratification at risk. Ultimately, it puts the responsibility of defining self-identity in the hands of people with whom we have had little to no contact. Yes, we want to be liked, we want to be loved, but there are no safe ways to achieve what we so desperately desire which, in the end, is intimacy.

True intimacy cannot be found in an ideology or group identity, for in those you are not an individual, you are merely a compliant member of a greater number of complying members. Intimacy at its core is terrifying. It is a definitive trigger for anxiety. Intimacy requires us to disrobe our defenses in moments that our anxious minds deem as high risk. If we risk, by default, we face the possibility of failure, embarrassment, and full exposure in the full glory of our weakness and fear. Yet, deep inside the recesses of our minds, this is what we are hardwired to seek out. Somewhere in the translation, we develop complex coping strategies and social constructs that protect our vulnerability and ultimately undermine the very thing we desire in the name of self-preservation.

The anxious mind races around every scenario of social interaction. The more adept the mind, the more processing is involved. 'If I say this, I will look foolish.' 'The way this person is looking at me tells me that they are not interested in knowing me.' Thought after thought races and in a moment's time, we are filled with innumerous questions and the panic is triggered. The anxious mind tells us that we are tired, or that we need to do something else. We will cancel outings with friends, limit our interactions, avoid going to noisy public places, eventually this urges to avoid progress, and in a very likely manner, we will develop debilitating phobias.

All of these things occur because we are faced with an existential conflict in one or more central areas of our life. As Yalom pointed out, there are four main existential categories, perdurance, groundedness, community, and pattern. If we were to take a strictly environmental view of life, we would see endless streams of data telling us that we are in conflict with these central existential categories. Yet, we still function with the presupposition that there is no conflict, or we minimize the magnitude that each existential conflict produces. One example of this would be that many bookstores are filled with aisle after aisle of books on self-worth, self-improvement, and pragmatic guides to life. There are entire sections called self-help. This is to suggest that the self can help itself. We find on other aisles books on motivation, calendars with motivational quotes. All of this to say that we know something is wrong and it terrifies us to the point that opposed to doing the dirty work of true critical-thinking, we would rather have someone else experience it, sum it up, and simplify it. It is not that the intelligence is lacking, it is rather that the heart is tired, aching, and anxious. If we open Pandora's Box, we can never close it. Once we peer into the depth of meaningfulness and groundedness, we are forced to look at the contrary categories of meaninglessness and groundlessness. If we look deeply into the category of community, we must ask what it means to truly be known, and what it means to be lonely. We must face the bold truth that many of our own coping strategies achieve polar opposite results of these foundational and existential categories, and with this knowledge, we are left defenseless and anxious.

So, why do we crave so deeply for these categories and why do we sabotage the fulfillment of them as well? There is a propensity within all of us to want to be good enough, to be desirable enough. Marketing strategies often focus on these fears. I would challenge you to watch advertisements from the following perspective:

1. Advertisements directed toward men often show a strong man, confident, desirable, and capable. This is why professional athletes are paid tremendous amounts of money to stand with a product for thirty seconds or to wear their brand of shoes, clothing or equipment.

2. Advertisements directed toward women will justify the need for a product in the fact that it will make the user socially fashionable, desirable, and ultimately, more attractive. This is outrageous as it reduces existential needs to appearance and acceptance by the general populous as the ultimate measure of purpose.

When there is so much outrage over sexism, and the debate of equality is always raging, we rarely hear much in regards to the generalizing and subjective means of minimizing the existential roles of gender to sell a product. Why? Because at the core of our being, somewhere buried deep down, we want it to be that easy. We want the solution laid out before us in a way that allows us to incur the least amount of pain and struggle. We do not want to experience fear, emptiness, or loss. We want to change, but at what cost? Recently, I was having a conversation with a friend. We were talking about the process of change. How do we change? Why do we change? At one point, my friend asked me, "Jason, you are a therapist, what do you think makes people change?" Firstly, I know that when a question is prefaced with, 'you're a therapist,' it really means, 'you are crazy enough to live in the deep end of the pool, what's that bottom like?' My response was simply this, "Nobody wakes up in the morning, experiences a wonderful day, and after speculating the immense beauty and a splendor a wonderful day offers, turns and says, 'No, this is too wonderful, I want to change this.'"

As a matter of fact, it is the absolute opposite. We do not want one thing to change. It is only when we experience some essence of suffering, pain, or loss, that we begin to process that we may need to change.

So, now, we are left at a critical juncture. If change comes through these means and we fear the very thought of them, why would we not sabotage the existential longings? Would it not be better to live in a constant state of oblivion convinced of an ideologue that promotes beauty and strength along with elegance and competence? The truth is that we desperately try to live in this world, but the more we remove the depth of an individual's identity and lay it at the feet of an ideologue, we create a much deeper sense of craving. This is because we are creating a false narrative. We are creating a storyline that sounds wonderful and amazing, but on the inside, is festering with fear and insecurity. The Zeitgeist of the day is one of intense individuality, as long as it is within the greater confines of the group identity. Social forums are filled with selfies. Picture after picture is filtered and re-filtered until it produces just the right image of who we want to see and be seen. We crave acceptance without risk, intimacy without the fear of rejection, being known on our own terms, and ultimately, it becomes isolation from the world. I am reminded of the great and powerful Oz in the movie, *The Wizard of Oz*. Upon first encounter, the wizard was greatly feared as he presented an image of himself that was terrifying. That is until the curtain was pulled away, revealing only a simple man. It was only when he was exposed, that he was able to change. It was at the moment when his coping strategy was literally pulled away, that he was finally experienced in the community, not as the powerful Oz, no, just as a simple man. He was known, and I would posit that this would be the fulfillment of a great existential need.

Chapter 5
Anxious Freedom

The anxious mind is one of constant motion. It does not rest well; it is always processing scenarios. This is, due to the fact, that anxiety is a state of feeling a loss of foundational control in some area. Anxiety is a combination of both chemical and environmental factors. It can have a predominately chemical causation or environmental, either of which can produce the same outcome. The duration, as well as the severity, can vary. Many experience panic and anxiety after a traumatic event, such as the loss of a loved one or a natural disaster, while others may experience childhood traumas from which anxiety manifests throughout their lives.

While anxiety can be debilitating, there is pattern. Each of us has triggers, things that cause our anxiety to rise. As we understand those triggers, we can begin to understand the origins of our anxiety. Many therapists will tell you that understanding your triggers is a way to stop your anxiety. There is some long-term truth to this notion, but not in the way that is necessarily intended. When we look at Cognitive Behavioral Therapy, for example, the emphasis tends to be on understanding your triggers and immediately changing the behavior surrounding it. The idea is that if you can master your habits and reactions, then in a short time, you will be free of anxiety. I find this to be a rather naïve understanding of how people change. This focus on control, which for some may have a short-term placebo effect, will eventually ebb by the wayside and the anxiety will return. This is because control, at least in this context, is a mirage. It does not exist. If anything, the long-term effects of this approach are more damaging because the coping skills that are taught do not begin to touch the surface of the true notion of control and will lead only to a hindered sense of true freedom.

So then, what is true freedom? Can it be obtained and felt? Before we begin to talk about what freedom is, let us first discuss what it is not. Every individual must struggle with certain desires and realities. There is a longing for a sense of belonging, a sense of meaning and purpose, and hope. When an individual avoids the negative correspondents of these, then they never truly struggle. It is a world of hiding and creating, creating measurable outcomes that reassure that there is control. When the world is approached from this perspective, there is little room for catastrophe, hopelessness, meaninglessness, and loneliness; that is, until it is forced upon us by some event or situation that shows our sense of control as the mirage that it has become. Freedom then cannot simply be a grasp of avoiding negative influences nor can it be denying the darker sides of ourselves that the mask hides. If this is deemed as freedom, it is short-lived, and one is left only with the responsibility of grounding an entire world under the pretenses of positive affirmations and a shortsighted sense of completeness. Responsibility becomes the coping mechanism for minds that have not embraced the world as it is, both positive and negative, both light and dark. The same can be said for an individual's understanding of themselves. We grasp responsibility because we cannot handle freedom.

Supposing that an individual can embrace that they are both dark and light, that they are both a sense of angel and demon, could one experience true freedom? This would mean that freedom is not contained in a single category. It is, at this point, that the treacherous cycle of anxiety begins to rear its head. It is here that an individual, deep within the recesses of their mind, will grasp the worst-case scenario of themselves and this, this is what they will believe; the entire time, they are showing the opposite reality to the world around them. They are grasping at this external sense of control, the mask, which allows them moments of clarity. This mask or Persona, nonetheless, is an integral part of every individual.

The Persona is that part of ourselves which the world sees. It is, in a healthy form, the desire to fit in with the world around, to leave a good impression, and to be equipped to achieve societal norms and roles. The Persona also serves as a Segway between the deeper parts of our lives. Imagine two individuals meet in passing. They begin a topical conversation. Perhaps, they find that there are shared interests between them, or maybe they present a similar sense of humor or style of communication. They are experiencing the Persona of the other. As the mind perceives that this person is safe, simple trusts are built. They may begin to talk about more central interests. Over time, as a friendship grows, they may share intimate details of themselves. They have moved beyond sharing the Persona and have moved to a much deeper and less defensive place in their friendship. The Persona has thus, served as a segue communicating to each that the other is within a certain norm or rather, a preferred norm that is safe.

The dark side of the Persona does much the opposite. It creates a false impression of the deeper self. It serves on one hand to protect the shadow side of the individual, and on the other, it serves to provide a false sense of control by manipulating the world around the individual. This is done creating a false sense of reality around who the individual is; it is a mirage which serves as a distraction from the shadow side. The anxious mind with its swirls of insecurities and fears unwittingly gravitates toward this. I have spent roughly 45,000 hours in sessions working with many individuals, and in that time, I have seen very few who are aware of this false Persona. It acts as more of a defense mechanism. Possibly, it is an internal conversation that might sound something like this:

"I am trying so hard to be okay. I don't know what to say at parties or around friends. I see what others say, and it sounds so much different than what I think or feel. I don't like this feeling of never quite fitting in. I want to fit in. I want to be good, at least, good enough to be loved or even liked. I want to be able to just hang out and not worry about every detail of what every person in the room is thinking or feeling, but it just seems that I'm always alone, even in a room full of people. Maybe if I learn to talk about the things that those around me like; maybe if I just say the right words and look a little less nervous, then I can fit in. Perhaps, not for long, but at least for a few moments."

Thus, the anxious mind works its magic, and a false persona is created. It can be quite effective, and many people will see it as honest and safe, but beneath the Persona is the continual anxiety, the constant questioning, and the fear of intimacy and trust. Ultimately, the false Persona, as it stands, will always face the deepest rejection. As intimacy and trust begin to develop in the midst of the false Persona, a shocking reality begins to dawn on the anxious mind. This reality is that there is a big difference between who they have tried to be and who they truly are.

The problem is not due to a lack of effort, rather, it has more to do with a lack of awareness. 'Who am I?' is one of the toughest and most challenging questions that we will continue to answer throughout our lives and when compounded with anxiety and depression, it becomes even more difficult.

It is incredibly challenging to discuss authenticity without a sense of awareness. There are countless ways to measure awareness. Descartes, a philosopher and mathematician, penned the term, *'Cogito ergo sum,'* meaning, 'I think, therefore, I exist.' Descartes set out on an epistemological journey. He wanted to get to the base level of what we know and how we know it. He began to eliminate everything that was questionable. He removed each and every variable systematically until he was only left with the fact that the awareness of his own existence was the only undeniable claim that he could make. Now, the average individual does not question the core of existence, as a matter of fact, the vast majority of the population tends toward a pragmatic mindset. To put it simply, we do not question why something is; we question how to use it. We live in a society that requires immediate gratification, and there is no time to stop and question the why's of life. We take life in chunks and broad categories. Those categories tend to be the receptacles for most of our understanding of the world around us, as well as ourselves.

Why take pragmatism over thorough and deep questioning? Pragmatism produces results, it offers a quick framework for accomplishment, and a sense of purpose, belonging, and meaning. We choose shorter condensed versions of experience. This rush for completion and gratification leads to a great lack of patience and self-awareness. This is truly one of the biggest contributors to anxiety, as well as depression. This is connected to great strides in technology which have allowed us to accomplish much more in a shorter period of time. It was only a couple of decades ago that the majority of our information was conveyed at an incredibly slower pace. If we go further back to the beginning of the last century, it was exponentially slower. There were more conversations and community held a much more direct place in culture. This is not to say that earlier generations didn't have that share of troubles. It was in the 1900s that we saw two World Wars, the Korean War, Vietnam, and the first Gulf War. As information increases its volume and pace, it forces societies and cultures to adapt and with adaptation, comes a change in the pace of life.

Society has changed more rapidly in the last century than all other centuries combined. We have adopted a pace of life that is so much faster, a world where information is more readily available than at any other point in history, but at what cost have these great strides come?

When the pace of societies increases so quickly, it is accompanied by constantly shifting norms. Fads come and go so quickly, it requires constant attention to keep up with them. We have become a society chasing our identity, an identity that has been externalized to the point that there is very little focus on the internal identity. Any time, self-awareness is sacrificed for a strictly externalized persona; intimacy is lost. Since the 1950s, the divorce rate has increased to the point that fewer marriages succeed than fail. The average age of marriage has increased as well. This, I believe, is tied to the fact that marriage is based on intimacy. Often times, we use the word vulnerability when referring to intimacy. This is such an odd term as in any other context, it has a negative connotation. When we refer to the vulnerability of soldiers' armor, we are talking about a weak point that if exposed in battle, it can be the cause of serious injury or even death, yet, we still link the term to intimacy. I would say that the connection becomes very obvious when we observe intimacy in marriage. Intimacy, in this context, is a commitment to living without defense. When your spouse says something that triggers your insecurity and anger, it is because they know your faults, your weaknesses, insecurities, in short, they know where you are the most vulnerable. This leaves many perplexed and hurt. When we lay our vulnerability at the feet of our spouses, friends, or family, we are trusting that it will be recognized and handled with the greatest care. Sadly, this is not always the case. Vulnerability; access to both the persona and the darkness that lies beneath is a risk. Every person has a shadow side, and we will experience betrayal, pain, loss; it is only through a healthy sense of self-awareness that we may gain confidence in dealing with the risk of intimacy. If I have not embraced the darker side of who I am, I will clothe it with shame and hide it away. When it is exposed, I will experience embarrassment and shame on new levels. This is because we actually believe that we are in control. The fast-paced world teaches us that we must always be in control, always aware of everything around us but neglecting everything within us. The gap between the persona and the inner-self has expanded more and more, leaving little room for true intimacy and a wide berth for insecurity, anxiety, fear, disappointment, and sadness. Is it surprising that there are so many apps developed to edit your image? Selfies have been around for quite a while and with them has come an unlimited world of options to hide every flaw and blemish. We can make ourselves appear younger, thinner, darker, lighter, and so on, to the point that a selfie is no longer about the self. It has become a polished, touched, and retouched image of the person we want the world to see. We have distorted beauty to the point that it no longer exists naturally and is never quite good enough. We have redefined the term to the point that it could literally mean beauty is you (with a lot of help). If our persona, our outward appearance to the world is no longer good enough, then what must this say about the inner-self. The part of you that you think is uniquely flawed to the point that if anyone ever saw it, they would run and never look back. We have created so many layers to hide this shadow side, and yet, this is where the greatest hope for intimacy exists.

We have praised external accomplishments to the point that internal accomplishments are not even a consideration. There is more to you than the image that the world sees. There is a treasure in your awkward faults. Intimacy is awkward, and so it should be, but over time, as we expose the darkness within us, it no longer has power over us like it once did. The anxious mind will tell you that this is dangerous, and it will be counter-intuitive. You may see the dark part of you as untouchable and unlovable. You may think that your mess is different and so much worse than anyone else's, but rest, we are all a piece of the same mess, and everyone who has an ounce of awareness has a basic instinct to hide the exposed and broken sides of themselves. Vulnerability in relationships is just as dangerous as vulnerability in war. Choosing to be vulnerable is not weakness, it is the bravery that would propel a soldier to run into battle, knowing that every defense has its vulnerability. Anxiety will tell you to run, to get away, to isolate, and it feels freeing to run from the things that terrify us, but is this freedom? You are free to be, free to be both mask and mess; you are free.

Freedom generally has great connotations, but the reality of freedom is that it is not always what it seems. As a matter of fact, the responsibility of freedom will lead many to limitations of freedom, whether on an individual level, or a societal level. This is not to say that limitations are unnecessary, as laws themselves are an agreement of limitations to protect more fundamental freedoms. However, we will focus more on the individual's avoidance of freedom in the context of this discussion. The anxious mind functions on limits. After all, the illusion of control can only be deemed successful based upon one's ability to limit the effects of environmental variables which can trigger greater anxiety.

Each choice we make is a limit to its antithetical counterpart and the anxious mind by physical necessity functions on a system of thesis and antithesis; for example, fight-or-flight responses. Marsha Linehan, in her work with Dialectical Behavioral Therapy, has championed the field of synthesis between black-and-white thinking. Her work focuses primarily on the concept that an individual is not limited to only two options. This is the circle of logic that many mental-health disorders find their home.

Chapter 6
Hope, Reality, and Good Intentions

Several years ago, I was at an airport in India. As I waited for the boarding call, I saw a child. He was five or six years old, and just like any child his age, he had a combination of energy and an absence of inhibitions. He danced about freely, awkwardly, and strangely, there was no music. When he saw that I was watching, the performance became livelier. He jumped and wiggled as he laughed, each time looking over subtly to see if his audience was still engaged. As I saw this display of careless freedom, I began to think about when my carelessness and freedom had disappeared. I began to look around the terminal, and I noticed that no adults were dancing as a matter of fact. They all looked tired, rushed, and irritable. I imagined that I was in one or more of those categories too. I thought back to the last time that I danced, and as I collected the moments, I realized that they all involved alcohol. I even remember saying at one point, that I don't dance without drinking beforehand and yet, this child had all the freedom in the world. The airport was his stage, and he owned that stage. There was little rhythm or rhyme to his steps, and honestly, there really was no need for it. He was free; he was transparent. He wasn't trying to convince anyone that he was the best dancer in the world, he just danced.

Having an anxiety disorder, I tend to have limits that others without a disorder might not have. My anxiety can run rampantly at times, and I will entertain it. I will sit, worrying about things that seem on the outside to be quite absurd. I will dread activities, at times, to the point that I will avoid them entirely and yet, at other times, I can engage and function with ease. It becomes difficult to know what will trigger my anxious mind and thus, begins the dance of control. These are the moments that I refuse to embrace the idea that control is a construct of the mind that allows me to engage tasks and social activities. Control itself, as we often define it, is merely an illusion, and yet, when a fundamental comfort space is violated, we take up the mantle of control as if it were real and attainable. I will eliminate variables, things that threaten my sense of control. I may avoid a person or people altogether. I may decide to go grocery shopping at 2:00 a.m. to avoid crowds and loud noises. Whereas, ironically, I love public-speaking. It is this incongruous set of fears that makes my mind race, and I commit to the illusion of control. I avoid my reflection in mirrors because I hate my appearance. I avoid weighing myself because I'm self-conscious of my weight. I have even avoided doctors' appointments because I knew that I would be weighed by the nurse. Somewhere in all of this contriving, I lost my freedom to let go and enjoy the simple freedoms that a child enjoys without a second thought. Now let me be clear, I am not saying that we should be dancing in the airport, but I am saying that there is a carefree sense of freedom that we lose when we embrace control as a real entity.

We live in a world of good intentions. Even when we are wrong, we still maintain the idea that our intentions were good, and sometimes, they are. However, this is not always the case, and I would say it is probably more than we would like to admit. When we begin to break down our actions and our thoughts leading up to them, we become much more aware of the complexity of even the simplest of activities. One example would be a conversation, any conversation. Conversations are not merely an exchange of information, but they are also the expression of power. Every conversation functions in this way. Maybe it is the physical posture we assume. Perhaps, the tone of our words, maybe we are giving advice or taking it, however, it comes about as there is an exchange of a power dynamic. I used to spend a lot of time in coffee shops, and there was always, without fail, that guy. He would be sitting alone at a table, continually talking on his phone. He would be loud, and his conversations would consist of short commands such as, 'just sell,' 'just buy,' 'that was supposed to be delivered yesterday,' 'get on it.' He is the guy that everybody notices because he has, whether consciously or not, dominated the entire area around him and he is making it clear that he is an important man, at least in his own mind. Without engaging a single person in the entire coffee shop, he has communicated to every person present that he sees himself as a priority. This is his persona in action, and it is one that takes up a lot of space. To some, he may look important, to others, he may be seen as someone who is narcissistic and prefers an audience when he is administrating whatever business he is conducting. However you perceive him, he has used his tone, volume, and general presence to dominate that space. Again, this is the persona that he presents, but beyond what we see, who is he? This is, in many ways, the design of an unhealthy persona; it is a distraction from the person. It is a façade that can be produced at any moment and can absorb a lot of power by sheer dominance.

Self-awareness begins with questions. It may simply be, 'who am I?' Regarding the loud businessman, it maybe be asking, "How am I perceived?" As an individual begins to ask these questions, they must consider the impact that they have on the world around them, both good and bad. Self-awareness, in this sense, is both terrifying and freeing. It is the beginning of a new framework, a holistic picture synthesizing who I am, as well as how I want to be perceived, which is both conscious and unconscious. The conflict that erupts in many people involves a fear of being perceived as powerless, incompetent, or unimportant. Every individual engages this in a myriad of ways, and yet, there are many overlaps. While there are many approaches, the stimulus is the same. If I can embrace that, at times, I power up not to maintain a sense of leadership or strength, but rather to avoid being seen as irrelevant or unimportant, then I can begin to grasp certain basic needs.

There are generally four categories of basic needs: perdurance, groundedness, community, and pattern. We will use these categories as a starting point in discussing self-awareness. It is also necessary to understand that these categories are evident at a very young age, and are generally solidified through childhood. It is, therefore, the case that we will need to overlay some platform for childhood development in the process of this discussion.

Perdurance

Every person has a basic desire to live on, to continue. This desire is not only concerned with survival, but also includes a fear of dying. Religions around the world share many things in common, and one of these is the belief in an afterlife. It is the idea that after death, you will continue to exist in some form or the other. Woody Allen once said, "I'm not afraid of death; I just don't want to be there when it happens." We are surrounded by the reality that death is inevitable and yet, we desperately want to avoid it as long as possible. What keeps so many in denial? No matter how advanced medical treatment may become, it has not surpassed the grip of death. No one wants to die, but throughout the journey of life, we are faced with its inevitability. What does it mean to come to grips with these vastly opposing realities, honestly?

This reality conflicts directly with our need for perdurance. We desire continuation, persistence, but are faced with a finite existence. The anxious mind pushes back with fear, a fear of an inevitable end and a lack of control. Yet, within these existential moments, there is more opportunity to embrace a deep sense of awareness, much more than in times of security and safety. Change does not come through comfort; rather, it comes from desperation and fear. When we avoid the fears that challenge our deepest hopes and desires, we continue in a persistent loop which keeps the hope alive through mere illusions of control. There are no five-step programs or approaches that will allow for epistemological rebellion. This is a process, an undoing, which, in its finest moments, enables us to see ourselves and the world more closely in its reality, as opposed to the construct of our own centrality in a greater scheme of existence. It is in this regard that we are allowed to experience ourselves in true freedom without the constraints of coping mechanisms, which have served merely as blinders, allowing to focus on the practical tasks at hand. What if, fully understanding our limits, we could actually embrace a purpose in life that greatly surpasses the glass menagerie that we had formerly embraced?

This is not to negate a need for pragmatism; it is quite the contrary. It is only when we embrace things as they are, that we can even begin to adopt a true pragmatic sense of being. Otherwise, we are left to the constraints of a world that is fragile, unmovable, and an end in itself. It is through our own sense of suffering that we can begin to understand the suffering of those around us. Empathy is the ability to understand and even share the feelings of others. Empathy cannot exist if we are unaware of our own true, deep feelings. Embracing the fact that, at some point, every life ends at face value, sounds somewhat depressing. The anxious mind spins to uncontrollable speeds as images of loss flash before it. Loved ones who will move forward, events that will take place, laughs, smiles, hardships that will all continue which we will no longer be able to share; all of which pushes us to a greater unknown. Risk then becomes an escape from experiencing the greater reality as opposed to the freedom of experiencing its true fullness. The anxious mind will move more rapidly to a state of hopelessness and meaninglessness where it will spin until we either embrace the reality as it stands, creating a synthesis with our more profound desire, or find another coping mechanism which allows us to move through another day in a state of oblivion. This means that for the anxious mind, it must exist in a state of tension between a desire for control and a reality which seems to be contradictory to this desire. Thus, synthesis reframes what appears to be contradictory as paradoxical. The consideration that opposing ideas may, in some manner, be part of a higher function that has been left unfathomed by a fearful and anxious mind, allows for acceptance, growth, and forward movement. Elisabeth Kubler-Ross, who gained notoriety through her work on the process and stages of grief expressed this sentiment, "It's only when we truly know and understand that we have a limited time on earth – and that we have no way of knowing when our time is up – that we will begin to live each day to the fullest, as if it was the only one we had."

The anxious mind exists in antithetical terms, yes or no, fight or flight, life or death, and the list goes on. Taking a dialectic approach which involves more complex and often, more categories than two, requires the mind to move away from anxiety. This is a physiological movement. The limbic system was not designed for sustained contemplation and complex thought. Its function, regarding anxiety, is merely to determine what is or is not a threat, and to react accordingly. This process requires two states, threatening or non-threatening, and reaction rather than process. It is only when that something is deemed non-threatening, that the mind can begin to process and synthesize a new paradigm.

Self-awareness is a continual process, it is not achieved in 12 steps. Pop psychology thrives on clean cut and tidy steps. You will find book after book, promising seven steps to be a better person, employee, leader, spouse, etc. The glaring problem with this approach is that it confuses the roles, doing and being. While the intentions are good though simple, their aim is to focus on the practice with the assumption that it will change the being. This is remarkably problematic, for if the state of being is unaddressed as a foundational causality for behavior, then the rate of recidivism will be much higher. Individuals can perform differently for periods of time without shifting their basic understanding, but over time, they will return to old habits and routines, as these have served in the past to quell both anxiety and insecurity. This is seen in the recreation of families of origin through marriage and the majority of addiction-recovery programs.

Though the intentions of such programs are good, the methodology leaves much to be desired and leaves the individual in a constant state of flux between living outside of a paradigm, which has been developed over the course of their lifetime, and externalized program, which functions on the change of behavior. The power of ambivalence in such circumstances leads to anger, frustration, to shame, and eventually, to isolation. The state of isolation most often marks a return to old habits and actions. Rearranging the deck chairs on the Titanic may change the appearance, but not the reality of the chaos which has ensued below the surface.

Self-awareness becomes a key element. It is not a simple task; it requires the individual to face realities which bear striking interruptions to the basic desires of the individual, as we have seen and will see in the following chapters.

It is only when the mind can grapple with the need for change that it can embrace the change that is required and this comes only through a greater awareness of the self.

Chapter 7
Security and Grounding

The anxious mind develops due to the perception of some conflict or obstruction from the four categories laid out in an earlier chapter: perdurance, groundedness, community, and pattern. This perceived or realized deviation is directly proportional to the gravity or base need for the fulfillment of these categories. In addition, it is complicated by the fact that understanding is both objective, as well as subjective. This means that an object itself is a source of data, in that it contains information which is indicative of the nature of the object itself. The subjective is the internalization or perception of the data based upon one's past experiences. It is the reason, for example, that when repairing an object, one often needs a tool, a screwdriver, for instance. While we may be unable to locate the tool, we find that a kitchen knife may serve the same purpose. The knife itself is what it is and contains only that information. Subjective understanding conceives that a knife may serve as a substitute for the screwdriver. This is based on the purpose of the knife, which may be adjusted due to the interpretation of the similarities of the objects. Thus, the summation of the purpose to fulfill the need for a tool. Hence, the screwdriver, while it is an object, becomes a symbol of something which serves a purpose and thus, the potential for a knife to serve as the embodiment or substitute for the symbol of a screwdriver, is realized. Perception and objectivity are therefore, interdependent for the further understanding and actualization of a symbol and substitutionary device or situation. This is a vague allusion to Plato's world of forms and thus, exemplifies the individual's inability to experience the full independence of objective reality, as all means of perception by default are based upon subjective methods.

This dichotomy is important as when we discuss the environmental triggers for anxiety, we must include the individual's subject experience as the sole means of perceiving the trigger as anxiety provoking. Any object or situation absent of the individual's perception cannot be considered anxiety-provoking simply because an object has potential data and unless it is realized, it will remain prospective.

This is not to say that the value of the object or individual is lost, instead, that it continues to exist, but is unknown. Melanie Klein, who was noted with Object Relations Theory, stated her observation of the interaction between external and internal, or subject and object:

I believe that the ego is incapable of splitting the object – internal and external – without a corresponding splitting taking place within the ego.

Though each person is cognizant, they are still a form of potential data to be experienced and perceived. I say this merely to lay the foundation for the complexity of relationships. The dynamics between two individuals include not only one perceiving the other, but rather, both perceiving and exhibiting data. This means that engaging and perceiving is continuously in flux, and therefore, misrepresentation and misinterpretation is common.

As I mentioned earlier, every individual exhibits a persona or mask. If we look at the mask through an objective and subjective lens, the mask serves to provide desirable data. This is a natural part of human experience and is tied to self-preservation and the need for community. Hence, if the mask presented negative or undesirable data, it would serve to sabotage potential acceptance and would show a deviation from the societal norms. Therefore, the persona serves as a filter between the outside world and what is repressed below the surface. This can serve a healthy purpose in the sense that it conveys awareness of societal norms, and thus, serves to communicate a desire for intimacy and community.

The Shadow and the Persona at odds (A will to power)

The complexity of interactions between two objects, which are also subjective perceivers, means that both can display the most desired data to be perceived. This may serve as both to initiate intimacy, as well as sever relationships that are observed to be of some intrinsic danger. As is often the case, when there is an emphasis on the persona, there is either unintentional or willful repression of the Shadow. It may simply be that the individual is unaware of the repression and has thus, become detached from the Shadow itself. Sufficed to say that willful repression or naivety ultimately serve the same purpose. This disconnection between the Shadow and the persona is a split in the ego, as previously stated by Klein. When a divide between the Shadow and the persona occurs, the individual will compensate for the discrepancy of reality and desire through the act of ambivalence. Thus, the traits of the Shadow will initially be projected outward. This projection provides an externalized method for the individual to confront the repressed internal side. The persona will serve once again as a barrier to the undesired traits by means of severing ties or passing judgment on the externalized recipient of the projection. This reactive stance is derived from the region of the mind which maintains self-preservation or continuation as perceived by the individual, but this perception is skewed due to a disconnection between the Shadow and the Persona and hence, the ego.

Though community is desired by the individual, the balance and regulation between the Shadow and the Persona is responding to webs of multiple reciprocities, and thus, either a will to power or will to compassion is born. This antithetical construct functions in unison with the outworking of the disconnected shadow and persona. The Shadow seeks to be seen as the Persona wants to repress. It is in this context that the Shadow perceives that which the Persona cannot in its current state. In order to achieve a true sense of community, it is necessary to be known beyond the Persona to the point of reconciliation with the Shadow.

Interpersonal relationships are an extension of the same process. The more intimate the relationship, the more necessary the need for individual development in the forming of tension between the Persona and the Shadow. This is evident, for example, in marriage. It is often the case that one partner will have a stronger perception of the external world. Therefore, one will have a tendency toward the complexity of appearance within the surrounding community, while the other will have a tendency toward isolation, hence a simplified view of external perception. When a lack of balance or tension exists within the individual between the Persona and the Shadow, it will be carried forward as conflict and perceived as a lack of validation or effort from the other partner. This discrepancy will be projected and will have a direct impact on the relationship. Manifested by a misinterpretation of the symbol of Persona or Shadow as a threat rather than a complementing component, one needing the other for the completion of a common expression and experience of realized intimacy.

The Shadow and the Persona in Love (A will to compassion)

Where congruity exists in a relationship between these points, the beneficial necessity is recognized as a completion of either the internal or external perspective and is, therefore, valued for this quality, as opposed to being perceived as a threat and rejected. Thus exists a need for a common conception of the two at work for one purpose, though vastly different, but complementary.

The anxious mind will perceive a partner as the trigger of insecurity through the relationship where anxiety is expressed and experienced. However, the partner is merely a projected symbol of the perception of the internal conflict; hence, anxiety is not based upon an external trigger, but an internal perception of a symbol as a threat.

The work of the anxious mind is often done in black and white, fight or flight, and is lacking the ability to develop synthesis. This inability re-establishes an emphasis on an antithetical dichotomy in which a deep sense of insecurity or incongruity between the basic needs of the individual for security are juxtaposed to the risk of intimacy, as intimacy requires risk and dialectic potential.

The anxious mind will retreat from intimacy much in correlation with the fight-or-flight response as the symbol of intimacy, in this case, the spouse represents a threat to the distorted tension or coping mechanism developed by the anxious mind. The term vulnerability has negative connotations and is often used synonymously with intimacy, i.e. a vulnerability in armor. The anxious mind perceives intimacy very much the same way, and therefore, the process of intimacy is more likened to a battlefield and survival than a coming together in a synthesis of two perceptions as complementary.

The work of intimacy must begin internally with the misconceptions which have been established by past experience. The past experiences of intimacy, such as childhood trauma at the hands of an abusive parent, serve to create the symbol of Persona or Shadow; a construct of opposition. Therefore, the need for validation will only come via the conquering of the oppressing symbol. If a spouse is the presenting symbol, the need for validation will override the need for intimacy, and thus, a conflict is born.

The repressed need for validation, however, can only be conquered through the reconciliation of the symbol as not only non-threatening, but separate and categorically differing from the previous experience. A cognitive reframing of these categories must, therefore, be undertaken, and since this repressed fear exists in shadow, the expressive ability of the persona is necessary to bring the shadow to light. This concept, by all means, will be counter-intuitive. The anxious mind as the perception and association of exposure and vulnerability has been deemed as the undoing or loss of self. Instead, the synthesis of the individual, through these means, is the beginning of true self-realization; not undoing.

Through the cognitive restructuring of need and latent unmet need, the act of willful vulnerability allows for synthesizing the partner as a complementing component. Thus, freeing the individual from the battle, in Nietzschean terms, of a will to power, and liberating them with a will to compassion.

Perception functions in a series of repeated patterns or categories. The more repetitive an experience, either positive or negative, the anxious mind will perceive it as truth. This restricts the inherent and independent objective value of an individual. In other words, the reliance upon past experience must dictate the interpretation of the present and the conception of the future. The anxious mind finds much difficulty functioning in the moment, as it involved continuously in a cycle of predicting future threat based upon past experience. It becomes lost and disjointed from the present, thus inhibiting the realization of a current need apart from self-preservation. It is often the case that anxiety disorders are perceived as narcissism. This, however, is a misunderstanding of the presenting symptomology and the varying purposes of an 'externalized locus of control.'

The undoing of invulnerability at the hands of the threating symbol, however counter-intuitive it may be, is the greatest hope for the anxious mind, as it is on the battlefield of the will to power. The will to compassion is not a battle of will, but the surrender of defense and thus, the development of trust. This cannot be done in isolation. Intimacy can never function in a vacuum. The vacuum of isolation offers a retreat to the anxious mind, there are no variables in isolation so nothing is perceived as out of control. However, in this context, control is an illusion, a distorted symbol for the will to power. The will to power leads only to isolation, hence is the case that in all disorders, there is some form of isolation involved.

The fact that patterns are perceived from simplest forms offers the anxious mind an illusion that control functions in the simplest form, i.e. isolation.

The journey of the anxious mind to freedom is fraught with concepts of contradictory terms which are transformed to paradoxical opportunities for healthy tensions in constant flux. The anxious mind is looking for an endpoint of risk, in contradiction to continuous risk and balance, and will look for simple steps and answers as they offer a greater affirmation to the need for control or power. This, again, is represented in the multitudes of self-help approaches which provide simple solutions in the midst of isolation, all unconsciously appealing to the will to power over the will to compassion. This is also the case with Cognitive Behavioral Therapy which rose to prominence because of its focus on the tangibility of short-termed outcomes. C.B.T. is also accompanied with a lack of focus on the importance of the therapist-client relationship as a means of cognitively reframing the past perceptions of symbols.

Intimacy is terrifying to the anxious mind as it seeks self-preservation and safety, but sabotages itself at the hands of isolation, loss of meaning, and ultimately, loss of self.

There are no simple solutions or no quick fixes, only the continual journey toward self-realization, constant becoming, new perceptions of symbol, and the light of welcomed intimacy illuminating the path.

Part II
Ends and Means

"Act so as to treat people always as ends
in themselves, never as mere means."

— Immanuel Kant, *Groundwork of the
Metaphysics of Morals.*

Chapter 8
The Dilemma of Distraction

The path of the anxious mind toward awareness is continual, painful, and will exhaust every defense in our arsenals. It is, no wonder that it vacillates between states of fearful expectation and hopeless resignation. Emotional dysregulation is the hallmark of anxiety and is akin to bipolar disorder in this regard. Phases of hypomania pave the way for exhaustion and avoidance. Hyper-vigilance in its exhaustive fury reduces the individual to numbness and abandonment of passion. The perception of intimacy through this continually shifting lens is no less turbulent.

Intimacy requires patience, risk, defenselessness, consistency, and most importantly, transparency. Many schools of modern psychology focus on the consistency of the persona as a means of evidential persuasion to the subconscious. This is contradictory to the fact that self-perception is not based on a token system. Minor rewards for efforts to not change the perception of the anxious mind. Quite the contrary, the accomplishments of external effort which bear witness to the capability of the persona are eventually sabotaged by the very target of their aim. The external perception of one's progress will serve as a temporary salve to the need of affirmation, but the law of diminishing returns is an ever-present collector, and thus, the benefits of externalized efforts will lessen as the emotional need for affirmation grows. This is to be expected, as with any addiction, regardless of its origin, whether clinical or otherwise, will leave the consumer in a state of euphoria as endorphins and dopamine surge. In the end, dopamine and endorphin surges are countered by the brain's reductive tendencies to maintain homeostasis. The problem is never the symptom, it is on the other hand, that from which the symptom permeates. Yet, as the age of persona-seduction unfolds, this is its logical conclusion.

The stimulation of neurotransmitters as a means of cognitive reframing can be established in quick succession, to be precise, it is often the hook that draws a client to return after the first session. We call this the placebo effect. That is to say that in the first session of therapy, there is a direct correlation between the level of catharsis and the rise in dopamine, in short, it feels good to be heard. This should lead the practitioner, as well, to a much deeper level of awareness. Practitioners should be aware that these are typical responses to healthy catharsis, not a means of cognitive reframing. It is, therefore, the model of relationship worked out between therapist and client that stands at the threshold of change. One might ask, why would this be the next logical step? After all, do we not function in a culture that is driven by momentary glimpses of happiness and relief from our distress? Would it not be logical to provide a link between the short-lived experiences of happiness and peace of mind to provide the continual experience? If this were the case, then any number of substitutes would suffice for therapy, for example, if an individual receives affirmation through social media, a notification is delivered to the user, this notification produces a spike in dopamine. If one were to, as many already do, check each and every notification, there would be a need to make a more substantial presence on social media, thus continuing the chain of dopamine surges.

The continual emphasis of presence through posts, likes, and shares creates a greater responsibility until one is isolated from true forms of personal affirmation, and at great lengths, is drawn toward the perpetual exaltation of the persona, effectively isolating affirmation to the Shadow.

The Shadow desires to be seen, to be known, and experienced. This is the root issue. Hence, a continual underlying resentment of the Shadow for the Persona. If this were practiced in any relationship, it would be disastrous. If a spouse finds pleasure in their own furtherance at the cost of the other, resentment would fester from the inside and would ultimately destroy the relationship. It is notable to reflect back to the notion that the relationship between the Persona and the Shadow is often projected outwardly toward intimate others. If this disjointed posturing of the Persona is a means to an end in the context of therapy, then, as well, it will end in disappointment.

The fears of the past century focused on a centralized government with growing control over the freedoms of the population. There was a genuine fear, as much of Europe had experienced its fruition during two World Wars. It produced an Orwellian fear of restriction and continual observation, with little to no tolerance for deviation from the demanded norm. The mantle of this fear is still carried by many conservatives and libertarians as manifested in the constant saber rattling of constitutional integrity. This paradigm is sufficiently prepared for an enemy armed with weapons, bullets, and fascism, but what if this was not the true enemy. There are no book burnings, no restriction to information, and the conservative ideologue is one which most closely resembles what it fears. As a matter of fact, in the past century, the world has experienced an explosion in technology and information that has not been seen in any other time in history. We are bombarded with information; we are entertained without restraint, to the point that not only are we not outraged by restriction, we are numbed by overstimulation. I would say that we are living out the reality more attuned to Aldous Huxley, who penned these words in 1927:

"In the past, most people never got a chance of fully satisfying this appetite. They might long for distractions, but the distractions were not provided. Christmas came but once a year, feasts were 'solemn and rare,' there were few readers and very little to read, and the nearest approach to a neighborhood movie theater was the parish church, where the performances, though frequent, were somewhat monotonous. For conditions even remotely comparable to those now prevailing, we must return to imperial Rome, where the populace was kept in good humor by frequent, gratuitous doses of many kinds of entertainment – from poetical dramas to gladiatorial fights, from recitations of Virgil to all-out boxing, from concerts to military reviews and public executions. But, even in Rome, there was nothing like the non-stop distractions now provided by newspapers and magazines, by radio, television, and the cinema. In *Brave New World*, non-stop distractions of the most fascinating nature are deliberately used as instruments of policy, to prevent people from paying too much attention to the realities of the social and political situation. The other world of religion is different from the other world of entertainment, but they resemble one another in being most decidedly 'not of this world.' Both are distractions and, if lived in too continuously, both can become, in Marx's phrase, 'the opium of the people,' and so a threat to freedom. Only the vigilant can maintain their liberties, and only those who are constantly and intelligently on the spot can hope to govern themselves effectively by democratic procedures. A society, most of whose members spend a great part of their time not on the spot, not here and now, and in their calculable future, but somewhere else in the irrelevant other worlds of sport and soap opera, of mythology and metaphysical fantasy, will find it hard to resist the encroachments of those who would manipulate and control it." (Brave New World Revisited)

Awareness and reconciliation of the Shadow and the Persona are the starting point and as stated earlier, this cannot be done in isolation nor can it be done by stimulating that which is continually overstimulated. It is, at this point, that a central change must come. That centrality must embrace a substance which transcends the discontinuity of the Shadow and the Persona and not merely serve as a deterrent for awareness. When we discuss the therapeutic process, this must be addressed, otherwise, we will continue down the path of soothing symptomology at the cost of systemic losses.

Thus, the importance of the therapist-client relationship gains its relevance. What is meant by this term is that a meaningful exchange between both parties must take place. The client must experience an environment that is conducive for the Shadow to be seen and known, and the balance between Persona and Shadow experienced as manifested between the client and the therapist. While the setting of therapy is genuinely a manufactured environment, it must divert from manufacturing to expressing. This is necessary for that manufacturing produces an end product, while expression is a continual process. The aim of this expression is the synthesis of realities that exist but are differed in their perception through the Persona and the Shadow. The Shadow is feared because it is passionate, unpredictable, and sometimes inappropriate; it is that part of us that hungers and desires to create something more and it is the Persona which serves to filter and balance that urge to creation with pragmatic elegance. An expression solely from the Shadow would not provide intimacy to any furtherance than the sole expression of the Persona, but congruency presents the truest form of the individual, as it most accurately depicts the entirety of being. Hence, the development of the repressed Shadow is a necessity. When awareness is tempered by an agreement of the full ego as it exists, the perception of the individual's total needs is expressed not as an end, but a continuation. It is the expressed, always expressing in the act of constantly coming into being.

Not too long ago, during an interview, I was asked by a reporter, "How do you make a person change?" I was unclear whether they were asking: what is the catalyst of change or what is the process of change, so I asked for clarity. There was an anxious pause indicative of some sense of unpreparedness. This, of course, was not my goal, so I clarified, "Are you asking what makes a person change or what does change look like?" The answer was humorously simple, "Yes?" The problem is not that we are restricted from a coming into awareness, rather it is that we have collectively lost the categories by which we perceive and find it. I continued the interview by saying that, "Pain is the most common cause for change because it is that which we most avoid. Nobody wakes up in the morning fondly remembering a perfect yesterday and says, 'I cannot repeat that something has to change.' It is when we lose; it is when we understand that we are not what we thought we were, with a sense of despair, that we reach for something greater."

Sadly, the change that the vast majority of people reach for is that of distraction, as it is readily available and exists in a host of varieties. Why would they not? It is appealing, it offers promises of immediate gratification, and it appears controllable. The true value of distraction is that it is designed to pacify the persona. It provides a path of good intention that seems clean and clear of obstruction. This is appealing; it is digestible and simple. At what cost does such a change come? How can one become aware, prepared for true intimacy and yet, not have the foundational congruity of the very thing in which they avoid? Submission to distraction is a commitment to the avoidance of passion. Creativity is born in the Shadow, it is the Persona that offers to bring this creativity to reality. Distraction tears from us the suffering that, in its fullness, is the completely aware and creative self. Creativity is born in passion and passion as derived from the Latin, *pati*, from suffering. This is, not to say, that one should embrace masochism abandoning the pragmatic beauty of the persona, rather that one tempers the other and thus, the expression of awareness is born.

It is the therapeutic process that serves as a guide, mimicking the balance between the two nudging toward the Shadow or Persona throughout the process, establishing a rudimentary balance between chaos and order and thus, the therapeutic relationship establishes its pre-eminence.

The process of change, of awareness, does not come through the achievement of tangible data as proposed by many therapeutic forms. The process of change is merely that, a process. Tangible goals for the aware are not an issue as they become the symptom of awareness. Hence, progress is not measurable by mere outward action as many repeat mistakes and will continually struggle, but as awareness and balance come into frame, a profound understanding of the whys emerge. No longer is an individual a victim to naivety, but is introduced to the competence which had always existed but laid under the surface of compensation, and fear serving only as hope and potential, rather than actual awareness.

The anxious mind, as it learns to exist in the here, and now does not cease to be anxious. Instead, it is aware of why it is anxious, why it perceives the world as it does, but also, that this is not a limitation. It is an invitation to intimacy, to be known in its fullness as both beauty and mess. They no longer see themselves as a means to an end, but rather as an end in themselves. As one embraces an end in the self, it can finally be carried forward much the same way the repressed Shadow had projected its pathology on those closest to it. The value of self and others is actualized, and hence, the ability to treat others as ends in themselves and not as means is birthed.

Chapter 9
I Think; Therefore, I Am (A Mess)

The fragility of the human experience is remarkable in, that due to the complexity of subjective perception, a multitude of causations may be attributed to any one perceivable object. This is to say that it is possible to have multiple viewpoints of one experience due to the environmental history, genetic predisposition, and general potential for the individual to perceive. Thus, in the constant barrage of data, there exists an equally formidable number of relevant and rational approaches to define it. It is notable that across a population, there may be a shared understanding of data due to a shared environmental history. These moments of synchronicity serve as major influential factors in socialization, learning, and various levels of intimacy. The individual's subjective perception is also tempered with the presence of critical reasoning, and hence, it is worth noting that there are secondary and tertiary factors which contribute to one's overall perception of any one piece of data. These shared perceptions of synchronicity serve to facilitate, in some respects, one's place within a more significant number of individuals, hence, serving as a catalyst for defining the parameters of community. Historically, a community has served different purposes and as shared perceptions of existential needs are understood, a social contract is developed. This theory was laid out with much detail in John Stewart Mill's, *Utilitarianism*. The value of the individual within a community was determined by the level of attribution the individual offered to the continuation and sustenance of the greater culture. It is possible to effectively evaluate an individual in terms of their utility within a greater system, and in particular systems, this is a necessary process. For example, within a medieval community, if every individual possessed only the ability to build, there would exist the potential for great strides in structural complexity, but unless some portion of the population possessed the ability to successfully cultivate crops or to harvest raw materials for building, the culture would face its demise due to starvation and lack of shelter. Hence the over-arching dichotomy of potential and pragmatic action must be present for further continuation.

This, of course, is the macroscopic view of a discontinuity. It is necessary to understand that this occurs directly within each and every individual. Thus, there exists a battle between potentiality and actuality. One might ask, "Who am I?" I would posit that the response would be dependent upon the circumstance in which the question was posed. One might see themselves as an athlete, a professional, a parent, a child, a teacher, etc. I would say that these are, less sources of identity, and rather, forms of identification. Throughout history, humanity has erred and faltered in confusion between identity and identification. Identity may exist on several levels both in the conscious and unconscious mind; hence, self-discovery is littered with mistakes and fraught with a painful misconception of one's own identity. This is evident in the differentiation between guilt and shame. Guilt carries a connotation of action, for example, one may be guilty of cheating to win a game, and thus, the action is deemed negatively and as a violation of a societal or moral norm. Shame, however, is a label of identity in as much as one who is guilty sees themselves as an immoral or bad person. Identity gleamed through the lens of shame will determine that the only potentiality contained within the individual must be bad, and therefore, any action corresponding from that potentiality must be seen with similar disdain. This leads the individual toward a sense of identity based upon a coping strategy. This logic will lead to a disconnection between the individual and any responsibility of self-improvement, as there is no potential for improvement. It is a limitation that subconsciously confines the variability or uncontrollable nature of successful pursuits, in turn, eliminating the possibility of disappointment through failed attempts. Thus, the avoidance of disappointment serves to provide the illusion of control. If one deems themselves as only bad, then there is no disappointment of expectation, rather, only the reinforcement of the self-conceived sense of shame. It is a protective mechanism, a shelter from a perceived lack of control. Hence, the substrate paradigm is that of a will to power through sabotage.

The anxious mind has an immense propensity toward sabotage as a means of control and in turn, perpetuates a cycle of self-victimization. The manifestation of this self-victimization is often reinforced by well-intended gestures and words of sympathy for the individual's perceived identity. This produces a social construct which is fueled by an immediate sense of gratification through attention derived from self-sabotaging behavior. The long-term rationale will lead the individual to sabotage the relationships which offered the desired sympathy as a means of continuation to the perceived identity of shame. This perceived identity, instead, is an identification of one's fault as the totality of the individual.

The tendency of identification over identity can function as well in the form of self-importance. If one deems themselves as guilt-free and as strictly a positive contributor to the surrounding culture, the substrate belief functions, then to promote constant actions (as all actions are perceived as necessarily beneficial), thus reinforcing practical action over contemplation.

The construct of good versus evil, therefore, concerning identification over identity, to the anxious mind, becomes a mechanism in which the fight-or-flight response is evidenced. The anxious mind, when processing foundational or existential fears, has little ability to synthesize a tension between two antithetical propositions. Hence, it either identifies on one side or the other. This, again, is not identity, rather, identification with one piece of the antithetical construct. Either identification manifests sabotage and isolation, rather only the methodology differs.

This leads to a more profound conflict, not of good or bad, sufficient or insufficient, as these serve merely as detractors from the primary causality which stems from the illusion of control as a means of establishing the individual's sense of existential safety. Therefore, if anxiety is a reaction to a real or perceived threat, the limbic system functions to prepare the body to manifest a means of control, either through confronting or fleeing that which is perceived as being the threat. This is a necessary function when the threat which has been seen as an imminent threat. On the other hand, when the threat is perceived from a symbol of past threats, whether the symbol is representative of one threat or a culmination of previous threatening experiences, the body is prepared to face a threat which is merely represented fragmentary and out of context. When this occurs in any degree of severity, the flight-or-fight response is, as well, out of context. The heart rate increases, respiration rates change, acidity in the stomach increases, and the vast majority of neural functioning is dedicated to an antithetical construct of confrontation or avoidance. We call this a panic attack, as there is no external threat; only the manifestation of what is perceived from past experiences and assigned to an external stimulus.

This begs the question, if conception and perceptual accuracy function in opposing states, due to the complexity and vast layers of perceivable data and the internal assignment of identification over identity, then how does one truly define a sense of stability much less the means of control? Hence, I refer to the illusion of control. This is not to say that an individual does not exhibit any sense of control. One might say that when faced with a series of choices, the ability to choose one option over another is clearly a means of control, to which I would say, that while an individual does have the ability to make choices, those choices are markedly limited in their scope. An individual may choose to wear a blue shirt as opposed to a green shirt. Nonetheless, they are limited to wearing a shirt as social norms dictate that it is appropriate. If we say that it is the in the control of the individual to adhere to or violate this social norm, the question arises as to why blue over green? Is this independent of a particular bias due to previous experiences, whether positive or negative? It would be possible to continue this line of reasoning ad nauseam, and this simply reflects in the simplest choices; constructs of influence exist, whether based on externally perceived expectation, or of the internal conception of external response both negative and positive. Thus, even in the simplest means of establishing, an independent autonomy is thwarted at the hands of past experiences and future expectations.

Hence, we see both on a micro-social scale and macro-social scale, the importance and inevitable limitations of autonomic authority or control. The anxious mind will strive to rectify an alternative construct in which it will default to reactive measure, in other words, if a blue shirt offers the possibility of acceptance, then all shirts one wears will be blue. Adversely, if the social expectation is seen as undermining the identity of the individual, hence, delivering a negative connotation, then the construct will be that of eliminating all blue shirts and choosing to wear only green. This is state of flux between adoptive behaviors and those of rejection are reactive and thus, appear to the individual as a definitive source of control, but ultimately, are continuously tied to a vast number of influences. The conception of this overarching construct may be consciously or subconsciously understood. If consciously understood, the individual is aware that a decision is not, simply one act of choice, but rather, a series of options based on internal bias and desired external outcomes.

While the individual who may perceive this construct on a subconscious level, functions on the basis of reaction, disconnected from the conscious awareness of the complexity of control but, nonetheless, still exists within the boundaries of the construct.

It must be noted that in all circumstances, bias exists as a means of identification, whether in compliance or defiance. Ultimately, bias itself is a feature that reflects the nature of an antithetical construct. If, while driving, I choose to turn left, I have chosen left over right. Perhaps the bias offers a pragmatic and necessary function. It may be that in turning left, I am achieving a significant bias, maybe that of going to one's own home as opposed another's. These biases are tied to identification as they serve to achieve a goal in which one identifies as arriving at their own home. While the home may indeed belong to them, thus, they recognize it as their own, and perhaps it offers a sense of safety, pride, status, or achievement, they are not their home. Home is an identification: I may say, "I am a homeowner," and while this is true, they do indeed own the home, the substrate principle of identity is not contained in the identification of owning a home.

The anxious mind craves grounding. It desires a stopping place and thus, what it identifies as safe, it often recognizes as an extension of themselves, and the reactive fight-or-flight responses provide a means of establishing the sense of security of that stopping place. This is particularly evident in the fact that the anxious mind functions mostly in the future or the past, but does not thrive in the present. It is consumed with pouring over the data of past angst and future scenarios. It is in constant flux between the two poles and hence, does not live in the moment. At first glance, this appears to be a contradiction to pragmatic end, instead, upon more in-depth examination, we find that it functions for one sole purpose; safety. If one can fully understand the patterns and symbols of the past, it becomes easier to see them in the future. Those patterns and symbols which represent harm or threaten the continuance of the individual can be identified and either confronted or avoided. This would seem to be a logical conclusion as very few would identify with the desire to actively manifest negative consequences. The problem that the anxious mind faces in its vacillation between past and future is that it is ill-equipped to deal with the present. Hence, many of the symptoms of anxiety have a tendency toward some type of avoidant practice such as that of procrastination. As long as the event isn't immediate, it cannot serve as an immediate threat, thus allowing the anxious mind more time of safety, more time to prepare for the future deadline. We see this frequently in academic settings. An exam date may be listed on a syllabus which was distributed during the first day of a class. The anxious mind does not see the potential of immediate preparation; instead, it finds a sense of ease in the fact that it is not due immediately. While it finds a sense of peace, it also develops a sense of anxiety of the upcoming deadline. This anxiety will manifest increasingly in activities which serve to distract the focus of dread on the future event, thus complicating the ability of the individual to prepare for the deadline thoroughly. Logically, procrastination creates a more constant form of anxiety, as there is no forward movement toward the goal, but for the anxious mind, it creates a respite from engaging in the moment, it creates a form of control that says, "I do not have to do it now and therefore, it is not an imminent danger."

Those who struggle with deep anxiety are often accused of being lazy, slow, and undisciplined. Many therapists share the same view, but I see this as a profoundly flawed conclusion. The anxious mind must be extremely disciplined, processing information at a very intense rate, and the sustainability of constant reaction, while avoidant cannot be seen as lazy. It may be the case that the expected outcomes differ from those of a social norm, but this serves merely to show that prioritization for the anxious mind differs from that of a social norm, not that it does not exist.

Bias is necessary for any decision-making process. The problematic consequences of bias occur when that bias leans to an extremity which is disproportionate to the situational construct. That is to say; when an individual reacts to any given situation with a perceived sense of threat that exceeds the true nature of the situation, the reaction will be based upon the perception of the situation rather than the reality. Thus, the individual is interpreting symbols within the situation based on past experiences, and reacts to the symbols of the past. There are many accounts of soldiers returning from battle, struggling with post-traumatic disorder, experiencing extreme internal reactions to common external stimuli. They are not reacting to the present stimuli, instead, to what the stimuli as a symbol represents. This is a horrific experience as the mind is unable to map out the present accurately and thus, a disconnection from the present occurs. The immense pain and struggle this causes, reinforces the sense of danger in immediate symbols and thus, pushes the individual's awareness away from the moment.

Throughout this chapter, I have laid out the mess that being human contains. I have laid a premise that shows the extremely finite limits in which our sense of control functions and I have expounded the complexity of the simplest situations. This is a necessary process due to the fact that if we continue to function with a premise that offers control where control cannot exist, while it may produce a placebo effect, over time, it will succumb to the reality that control is attainable or achievable. The problem, in fact, is not control at all, it is the disconnection between the antithetical nature which exists between conception and action. If I reinforce the virtue of immediate control, I undermine the development of tension between the poles of conception and action. I will, ultimately, reinforce malicious habits which, without greater awareness, will simply reinforce and increase anxiety.

Chapter 10
The Depths of Chaos

The history of chaos and order has been recorded throughout history, from Greek Mythology to the present. We are faced with a protagonist which must struggle to face their own undoing and rise from the ashes with new strength, courage, and ability. This new creation is equipped to confront the protagonist.

Thus, the overarching theme is that when we face chaos, in this sense, which we do not know, there arises a new sense of order. A new degree of understanding which drives us forward to confront, once again, those things, which threaten to undo us.

If growth and change come from constant undoing and reordering, then why do we desperately avoid the undoing? I desire safety, order, security, and yet, to attain a greater sense of these things, I must dive into what feels unsafe, disorder, and no plan of securing my continuance. I would say that this would serve to contradict most individuals' definition of safety. Therefore, it is necessary to look more closely at chaos and what this journey truly entails.

Human experience serves as an invaluable resource to both predict future outcomes, to develop expectations, and to be prepared to succeed. Nobody sets out for failure, and yet, there it is, on every page of the human narrative, failure, suffering, and loss. The limits of our understanding often serve as the beginning of fear. This is why we project our expectations of an individual's persona on the individual and engage with our perception of them, until time and intimacy have developed. In turn, we deem it safe to allow ourselves to experience them in more of their own light. It is literally wired into the human brain to map out the past, and from the past, to map out the present and future. When we observe the structures of the brain, which there are many, but for the purpose of this book, we will look at two, the right and left hemispheres. The right hemisphere is designed to engage new experience; it is the source of creativity, it's wired to engage chaos, in essence, and it is the rebel of the neurological construct.

The left hemisphere, on the other hand, is hardwired for order, concrete logic, and rules. It is that part which is involved in pragmatic productivity. Left to their own devices, they would spin; the left hemisphere alone would be limited to the productivity of that which it has already developed rules and borders. It would never innovate, change, or vary, solely for the fact that to do any of these actions, it would require a deviation from what is concrete and known, in other words: chaos.

The right hemisphere alone would venture deeply into creativity, innovation, abstract reason, but could not serve to bring any of these to actuality as this would require order, rules, and a level of pragmatism.

Though the two function on antithetical terms, there is, in essence, a meeting of the minds. When data enters the brain, it is divided between the two hemispheres. Thus, two separate senses of consciousness are breaking down the data. As this process occurs, there is communication between the two hemispheres. Literally, neural pathways develop to establish a full concept of the abstract and concrete natures of data. One region may develop the pragmatic nature of what is, and the other, the possibility of what it might become. Therefore, the undoing of the protagonist and its renewal, or that which prepares it to emerge as a fuller, more aware individual, ready to experience greater victory, is constantly coming into being on levels that we are unaware.

There is, however, a propensity for the individual, whether due to environmental necessity or biological predisposition, to err more to one hemisphere or the other. In other words, there are those that cling to pragmatism and those that cling to chaos. This does not mean that both hemispheres are not at work, rather, that one is more developed and serves as a predominant basis for understanding.

There are those who read the instruction manuals to accomplish the task as it was intended to be and there are those who dismiss the manual altogether to create as they go. This is the source of much of the conflict in our worlds. When you are faced with an individual that craves only structure, and you crave the complexity which underpins the structure, one is viewed as unproductive and the other as inflexible.

These are patterns which are repeated on every level of humanity, from the inner struggle of the individual mind to the functions of couples, cultures, and nations. Hence, the pendulum between chaos and order is always moving to provide a counterbalance to the extremes expressed in each and every one of these realms.

When order is prevalent, it will remain prevalent until chaos has reached a fuller limit and must be addressed. Adversely, when chaos is predominant, it will remain so until there is an inevitable need for productivity and utilitarianism. Chaos appears to the ordered as the protagonist, as does order to the Chaos minded. The human mind is designed to separate the two and ultimately bring them together, creating a balance between innovation and productivity, chaos and order. Yet, when one errs too greatly to one side, the mind compensates by creating a supportive construct; this is what we refer to as a coping strategy. Coping strategies exist in multitudes; some being healthy and facilitative, while others serve as a means of continuing the imbalance. Reliance, on one without consideration of the other, produces a monster to which, in *Beyond Good and Evil*, Nietzsche says:

He who fights with monsters should be careful, lest he thereby, become a monster. And if thou gaze long into an abyss, the abyss will also gaze into thee.

In other words, avoidance of tension creates the most significant risk to the individual, thus, both chaos and order are necessary.

We have viewed the differences of chaos and order, and have established what appears to be a contradiction; I would suggest that rather than a contradiction, it may be considered in more paradoxical terms. It is not that the two are truly opposites, rather, two sides of the same coin. They are antithetical in function, but the function of each serves to feed the other.

It is generally at this point, that the anxious mind 'Cries havoc and lets slip the dogs of war.'

It contrives a means of order based on a panic response, which is based on yet, another antithetical system that is the limbic system. While the limbic system serves many purposes such as regulating involuntary processes such as heart rate, digestion, breathing, and sleeping, it also regulates the panic response which is fight-or-flight. Confront or flee, again the antithetical model appears. It serves, in this sense, to determine what provides the greatest means of immediate safety in an environment that is perceived to hold an immediate threat. Referring to a previous chapter, understanding the outside world is perceived through a projection of past experiences and conceived outcomes based upon those foundations. Thus, another tension between extremes exists, that of external realities as opposed to internalized perceptions of the outside world. We live in a world of objects or symbols full of potential data and yet, based upon the perception, we separate the dichotomy of object and symbol. Thus, if an object is perceived as a symbol of threat, regardless of its own independent potential data, it is, nonetheless, treated as a threat because symbolic means override independent attribution.

It is, at this point, the limbic system engages in contemplating the safest course of action. It is a system of black and white, fight or flight. This is the anxious mind at work, erring to one extreme as a means of securing the continuation of the individual which, again, is one of the foundational needs of human existence. The anxious mind, though, instead of contemplation defaults to reaction, it does not think it moves. It judges motives, intentions, and danger, assigning it to an object whether animate or inanimate, with high levels of prejudice. Or in Carl Jung's words, "Thinking is difficult. That's why most people judge."

When thrown into chaos, we instinctively look for order and patterns, as does the anxious mind. When thrown into order, we immediately move toward innovation. This is the balance of the mind working its way out. Just as the two hemispheres serve a separate purpose, there is a middle ground where tension exists. Fear is the variable factor that causes deep leaning to one over the other. We call this push from one to the other, ambivalence. Ambivalence is an amazing tool; it is an indicator of the internal need for balance, even in the midst of unconsciously ascribing the need to the self or the presenting situation.

The foundation for order and chaos itself, is based in the initial stages of life. These developmental stages are the first perceptions and conceptions of the world around and the potential that this world contains. Jean Piaget, who spent the majority of his career studying and identifying stages of childhood development, adds emphasis to this concept:

Before playing with his equals; the child is influenced by his parents. He is subjected from his cradle to a multiplicity of regulations, and even before language, he becomes conscious of certain obligations... The child of three or four is saturated with adult rules. His universe is dominated by the idea that things are as they ought to be, that everyone's actions conform to laws that are both physical and moral – in a word, that there is a universal order.

Children develop this universal order based upon their environment. They can only assume that what is around them is the order in which things should be, hence, when socialization occurs, that which differs from this order is viewed as chaos, serving to undermine the learned order of his or her family of origin. These interactions become more complex, as the complexity and depths of social interactions become more frequent. The interactions between chaos and order challenge the child to normalize either the norms of home, of their limited exposures with what differs, or to synthesize and normalize both. The importance of these primary, foundational norms serve as the basis with which the child will view what is order and what is chaos and thus, there is a tremendous dependence on the parent as a source of these norms. This is evidenced in Greek Mythology. Many myths focused on the demigods which were the offspring of a mortal parent and a god. Achilles was the son of Thetis and Peleus, Orion, the son of Poseidon and Euryale, Bellerophon, the son of Poseidon and Eurymedon, the nobility of the individual was founded in the elevation of the parent as a god. This is not only true in Greek Mythology, but is seen in Hindu Mythology as well; Arjuna was the son of Indra and Kunti, Bhishma, son of Shantanu and Ganga. The Romans were no exception, Bacchus was the son of Jupiter and Semele, Romulus was the son of Mars and Reah Silvia. This form of elevating a parent to the status through myth is common on some level in most cultures, including current culture which has created superheroes such as Thor and Wonder Woman, based upon their deified parents. It is of no wonder that the myth of the deified parent would exist so pervasively throughout culture and history, since myths have largely existed as a means of explaining that which was beyond understanding, through story.

It is also necessary to note that in each and every myth contains an epic; a becoming in which the protagonist comes into his or her own sense of self. There is a level of awareness achieved; an identity developed somewhere within the tension of order and chaos, it is this tension that elevates the protagonist to eventually embrace their destiny and to emerge victoriously. It is this great undoing which forces the protagonist to the very depths of their being; it is the necessary suffering that produces the greater being which had existed as potential, but emerged through the struggle.

If the parent remains as the only foundation of order, there becomes a total dependence of the individual upon the parent. In a non-religious sense, the deification of the parent, which outside of the context of the developmental stages of childhood, leaves the individual's potential unrealized. Meaning, the hero of that story has yet to succumb to the great undoing which establishes them as capable, competent, and aware. It is order which introduces the rules, the norms; it is the chaos which pushes the individual to a broken greatness which pushes the norms of order and chaos into tension, allowing them to not only function on norms, but also to embrace change and to compensate that tension to adapt, or as Jordan Petersons says, "That which can confront chaos and triumph."

Chapter 11
The Power of Woundedness

It is the wounded protagonist who has faced the ends of their original order which is forced to create something. Order without chaos has no variation, only a pragmatic function. Chaos without order produces possibilities without production. When order and chaos work in tension, there is forward movement, change, and newness. Thus, wounding is a force that destroys the previous nature of the relationship between one's perception of order and chaos. This previous perception had served as a sense of safety and a form of identity.

Les Miserable, a novel by Victor Hugo, follows the undoing of its protagonist. Jean Valjean, a man who was imprisoned for stealing bread for his starving sister, after serving nineteen years in the Bagne of Toulon, faces an uncertain future. Years of chaos had driven him to a much different perception of reality. Jean Valjean, after being turned away from one inn after another, finds refuge in the hands of Bishop Myriel. Valjean, hardened by the chaos of his past, stole the silverware from Myriel's home. The protagonist is apprehended by the inspector and is questioned in front of Myriel, to which he explains that the silverware was a gift and that in his rush, Valjean had forgotten to take the silver candlesticks. Myriel places them in the bag and after the departure of the inspector, instructs Valjean to take the money and invest them in making himself an honest man. The order in which Valjean had learned to live would have been chaos to most, the mercy shown by Myriel was a chaos that forced Valjean to reexamine what he truly perceived the world to be. Valjean, through many struggles, eventually establishes himself as a respectable man, but a man of virtue, able to show mercy, and equipped to navigate the chaos and order. Inspector Javert visits the now mayor of a town, Monsieur Madeleine (the alias used by Jean Valjean). After witnessing a great feat of strength by the mayor, he is reminded of only one man who would have possessed such strength, a prisoner which he knew in the Bagne of Toulon. His suspicion, fueled by his pursuit of law and order, leads to an eventual confrontation in which Valjean saves the life of the very man who pursues him. Javert inflexibly bent toward order, knows that as long as he lives, he must pursue Valjean. This inflexibility offers any deviation from the order which provides one path of logic: to free Valjean, Javert must take his own life. Valjean is spared, but the unmovable Javert followed the logical conclusion of order without the tension of chaos.

It was only through a great suffering, a loss of identification with the guilt and shame of imprisonment, and the label of a convict, and the merciful chaos of Myriel, that Valjean could begin the wounded journey of the protagonist. The ability to change, adapt, and embrace that which is beyond the illusion of control; these are the tools which equip the protagonist to embrace the actuality of his strength and the continual coming into being.

The anxious mind grapples with the tools of Javert, order, and control, in opposition to the antithetical chaos. It has no means of genuinely coping or embracing the chaos and is trapped in an endless cycle of shame, reinforced by the patterns of sabotage to maintain at least the sense of some identity, some sense of safety. The anxious mind will work, tirelessly examining scenarios attempting, out of context, to apply the rules of panic and continuation through reaction rather than engagement and synthesis.

The necessity of wounding is counter-intuitive. The idea that to come into one's own, one must meet a demise of the old self – goes against the very grain of the survival instinct. The language of suffering and wounding fly directly in the face of the majority of approaches in pop-psychology and self-help. We live in an age that teaches us to try harder, follow the steps, believe in yourself, and achieve. To introduce a form of self-destruction, much less an embrace of such a release sounds, at best, depressing. Is this perhaps because our modern, post-modern, and post-post-modern views have attempted to eliminate the process of necessary suffering, or at least, minimize it? Is it possible that we have lost sight of long-term goals and replaced them with immediate gratification? This, of course, comes with a beautiful marketed packaging. Can one grow without suffering? Has humanity come to a place where it no longer needs the voluminous accounts leaning to the contrary? Perhaps, this is more a testimony to the helplessness of the individual and a deep and aching for relief.

There is a long history of mythology and tragedies that if we follow them only to their demise, we are left wanting. What is it in the individual that continuously faces chaos and yet, is still disappointed when it becomes more evident, that chaos is not meant to be controlled? Again, the faltering point is built on the assumption that the choice is between order and chaos. I would suggest that order to one is another's chaos. This is more complicated by our internal perception and projections upon those around us. We are more than willing to assume that the world around us is somehow akin to having the answer, and that we are somehow on the outside, looking in, awkwardly waiting for the secret of survival and growth. This is the misleading message of so much of the work on self-help and pop-psychology. Change is not simple; it is not a leap from chaos to order, nor is it order to chaos. Instead, it is the realization that we are in a world of information which is in constant flux; one where there is, often, more need for chaos than order and vice-versa. There is a balance that looks less like a resting point and more like a journey which is unfolding before us, one in which we are the protagonist, and we are led by a host of predecessors which have been the protagonist in their own epic or tragedy. Even the Phoenix of Greek Mythology, no matter which variation of the myth one embraces, must face the fact that the brightest moments are a hint of a return to ashes, all so that it may rise again in its blazing glory from the dark ashes of its descent. As it has been said in the past, "It is always darkest before the dawn." To err toward chaos or order is a natural tendency, the push toward the embrace of both is where true fear exists.

Herman Melville captures the undoing of one individual in such loving detail, that it has remained a classic for over one-hundred-and-fifty years; that is the story of Moby Dick. The story is told from the perspective of a sailor named Ishmael. He unfolds the story of Captain Ahab's wounding and desperate need for retribution. Ahab, on a previous journey, had captained a ship which had suffered attack from a great white whale. In the midst of the attack, the whale took Ahab's leg from the knee down. Ahab had suffered a significant loss; he had seen the face of chaos and could reconcile any order from the chaos, hence, was driven by a desire to return upon the whale all of the injury and pain which he had suffered. This desire to return the pain which had been delivered, the concept that to force suffering upon the thing which has brought us suffering, ultimately, revenge, comes from a sense of unmet justice. This justice suggests an act of balance; what you have taken from me, I will take from you. Unfortunately, justice is not met in isolation, the subject of suffering is not an unbiased source to judge the means of balance. They are hurting, wounded, aching for the order in which they had once found comfort, in other words, they want a return to the old self. Unfortunately, suffering does not leave us the way in which we were discovered. Nonetheless, Ahab, unaware that he had been fundamentally changed was not able to embrace this change, at least, not in the sense that would lead him to grow. Ahab was driven, at any cost, to punish the great Moby Dick.

Melville: "He piled upon the whale's white hump the sum of all the general rage and hate felt by his whole race from Adam down; and then, as if his chest had been a mortar, he burst his hot heart's shell upon it."

This was not balance, nor was it an attempt of any form. This was fear, masked behind the secondary emotions of anger and rage. Secondary emotions are secondary, in that they are defense mechanisms which protect vulnerable emotions. Anger is a defense, one that is expressed in terms that are directly proportional to the fear, sadness, and disappointment, which exist below the surface. These are reactive emotions; they are meant to establish an immediate sense of safety and control in an adverse situation. Thus, when we act upon these secondary emotions, the logical outcome will be destructive, isolating, and ultimately, if left unchecked, will lead the story from epic to tragedy.

The anxious mind does not function in means of synthesis but much in the same way as anger, it operates in reaction to a stimulus. It distances, pushes away, eliminates variables, isolates, and if left unchecked or unengaged with some means of balance, will leave the vulnerable individual alone and more isolated than before. This is a source of deeper anxiety which functions, as previously stated, on the need for community.

The field of Mental Health tends to refer to normal and abnormal behaviors. What is meant by this is not that there is one particular place or dot on the map of behavior where normal exists, instead, normal is a range, an average, and this suggests that variations or movements within this range occur. It is as if there is a range of behavior between extremes, a tension if you will, between chaos in its totality, and order in its greatest inflexibility. Normality is not a fixed position and is not immovable, and must be viewed through the lens of multiple variables. When catastrophe strikes a community, or an entire society is affected by poverty and hunger, what would be considered societal norms, would be much different than a prosperous nation at a time of peace. The dance between chaos and anxiety is fraught with fear and awkwardness and yet, gilded with vibrant colors of love, risk, and loss. Fear drives the wounded heart to seek for safety in the repetitive nature of the past, a past that existed before the great wounds which present themselves through the forward path of life. The anxious mind will reel in agony as the past measures are no longer relevant. This is not because the pain is too great, not by any means, it is rather because the wounds deepen our desires and longings. It serves to take us to new depths in which the old and shallow coping strategies could never appease. Coping strategies lose their substantive properties in the face of reality.

As a child, one might find great comfort in the embrace of a cherished toy or stuffed animal, and as an adult, when embrace has found its center, not in a thing or a means to an end, but rather, an end in itself, in intimacy, the need for lifeless surrogate embrace can no longer compare in its width or depth.

Even the attempt to return to such strategies will drive an individual to further fears as they experience the fact that not even the best and the most developed surrogate can be no substitute for true embrace and intimacy. These fears arise when the mind suffers the loss of intimacy or its sense of security in the intimate other.

The necessary wounding does come, and even the best attempts to thwart its path fall short, as the undoing does not come from outside but from within. External circumstances serve as the stimulus which throws the internal balance off. What was normal and under control yesterday is no longer so. The individual must now struggle with a new realization that the world is not what it appeared to be. This undoing, a grieving that perpetuates something new, mature, and more aware.

The anxious mind is forced into a new reality with no mechanism for control, and just as it is designed, it reacts, it confronts, or avoids. It falters to unsustainable extremes. Therefore, the mind and the body cycle from anxiety, to exhaustion and depression, there is a deeper loss of ground and as that grounding is lost, fear escalates and anxiety returns. It is only that which is contradictory to the reactive mind, which will calm anxiety. It is the delicate dance between chaos and order, sometimes leaning more toward the edges of chaos but gracefully pulling back toward a new sense of order. This dance, this art form, is the expression of the wounded heart. The ability to show grace, mercy, and empathy only come from an experiential base of loss. Said loss, which frees the anxious mind, is the very loss that has the potential to perpetuate the cycle. Ahab was driven by woundedness to self-destruction, Jean Valjean was driven by chaos and after learning the intricate measures and steps of the dance, in the end, Valjean emerged as the wounded protagonist, fuller, more aware, and capable of mercy.

We are both Ahab and Jean Valjean, Myriel and Javert. The question we are left with is how do we dance between the extremes?

Chapter 12
Dancing in the Dark

The dance of tension does not begin with grace and ease; it starts with awareness. It is fascinating to me that the general opinion of counseling is that it is only for those with a serious problem. The reality is that it is only for those who are aware that they have serious issues, for we all have issues, we only differ on levels of acceptance and awareness. It is much easier to compensate and to push back from one extreme to the other, and as we have seen throughout history, this has often been the case. Whether in Literature, Politics, or Societal Customs, the pendulum is always in motion, and there are moments few and far between, but nonetheless, moments of synchronicity. There are times of peace, growth, and safety, and there have been times of great suffering, loss, and pain. It is the necessary suffering which surrounds us, which we all encounter, collectively and individually. The times of the most significant needs present the most significant innovations, which over time, send the pendulum in the opposite direction. It would seem that one norm prevails above all norms, and that is that of constant change.

The dance of tension is complex, shifting in moments from subtle movements, then abruptly to a rhythm of high intensity, and back again, sometimes, with no hint of predictability, yet the dance continues. Dance is a form of expression. If one dances to dance correctly to the system of one discipline then, at times, they will experience victorious triumph, until the inevitability of a changing rhythm occurs. It is, at this point, that the most talented of dancers would be ill-equipped, as the limits of the order of their discipline had been outreached. Those who would dance only to the tune of their heart, without an interest in any discipline, would find it difficult to find their place among the shifting beats and patterns. Only in the fleeting passionate moments of the dance that they would find their home. Those residing just in chaos, or strictly in order, may just dance intermittently and find frustration in the opposing moments, that is, until there is risk. What would the skilled, disciplined ballerina do if the practice led to improvisation, creativity, a letting go of the strictness of competency in performance, and an embrace in the passion of the moment mixed with the skill of an expert? The dance would be moving, maybe familiarly awkward at first, but nonetheless, moving and touching to both of opposing residence. What if, in the midst of an orchestral background of precision and order, the passionate dancer embraced the steps of the ballerina, not aside from their passion, but along with the freedom of chaos? Would this not enable them to embrace moments of structure and chaos paradoxically in a greater order, where rather than an antithetical pair, the two function as partners, in the dance itself?

This would be a sense of chaos and order for both; this is evident in marriage. A dance between two individuals functioning as one unit, still maintaining individual desires and needs which may go unmet by their dance partner. The dance may have moments of utter chaotic gyrations leading to moments of intimate embrace and graceful surrender, each acting in a counter-intuitive way to past experiences. This is the dance of tension in intimacy. It is a dance of risk, of hate and of passion, one of subtlety and one of aggression, appearing one moment to be as graceful as a ballet and the next, as chaotic as war. Over the years, the dance continues, based upon the risk of the individuals to invest in the chaos and order of the other. When a couple comes to therapy, it is usually due to some sense of weariness. Perhaps, one has danced with more intensity to compensate for the lack of the other. There is a breaking point where one will ask, "What am I getting out of this?" It is a dance move that often sparks deep insecurities in both, one feeling neglected while the other feeling overwhelmed with expectations. Defenses are built, walls which serve to misdirect the steps of the other, a dance of unpredictability occurs, achieving the exposure of the partner's inability to keep up or to stay in tune with the rhythm of intimacy.

Over time, if left unaddressed, then the dance, one which began with expectancy and joy, slows to a dance of expectation and grieving, solely for the fact that instead of dancing for each other, the focal point, whether in order or chaos, the dance returns to that of two individuals not in unison, but at odds, using the expression of their moves to establish a sense of comfort or power, and ultimately leading to a loss of desire for the dance.

It has been mentioned in earlier chapters that we function in a world of antithetical principles, springboards of escape from the intensity of one to the other. Couples generally seeking help have come in the midst of passionate chaos, and their dance is erratic and out of step. These are couples for whom the flames of love and passion have not fled, there is hope in love and hate for great strides, more passionate and unified than ever before.

However, there are couples that attend counseling long after the passion has fled. They appear tired, lifeless, only moving out of necessity. While there is hope in love and hate, there is little hope in apathy. The dance of grief has finished and a norm of separation has been established, and the only shared passion is that which maintains this separation. It is true that we will always dance, but whether it is a dance of loneliness or one of risk and passion, is restricted to an individual's ability and/or desire to defy the old norms. The constant flux of intimacy, much like the dance, requires the solid foundation of order and the flexibility and innovation of chaos. Intimacy is the place where order and chaos meet in a passionate kiss, as they dance for one another in a harmonious union.

Passion is more about the intensity of the emotion rather than a connotation to which emotion is expressed. Apathy is the absence of intensity, and inescapably the presence of desire left unexpressed and unmet. It is the breakdown of trust which, at some point, had been betrayed on one or multiple levels. It is the repetitive pattern of disappointment that leads expectancy down the path toward expectation.

Intimacy between two people means that there will be depths of love and shared experience, that each will be known in a new and passionate way. It also means that there will be hurt, hurt in the central and intimate places that once served to provide the very sense of closeness that now hangs in the balance. Anxiety pushes us toward self-preservation, to one of two extremes, those of confrontation or escape. Balance has pain and happiness as an underpinning for mercy and graciousness. It serves to remind both that as the experience of disappointment takes its grasp on the individual, that they also are aware of the faults within themselves, which have and will serve, to disappoint the other. It means that there is room to fail without shame, and to regain balance in partnership with one another, not in spite.

There is no roadmap for intimacy, and at many points in the dance, it will feel as if the lights have been turned off and now, there is only the feeling of a partner moving in unison and yet, still dancing; dancing in the dark.

Intimacy is counter-intuitive, in that, we are hardwired to crave community, and yet, when community threatens the need for a sense of perdurance, there is a conflict which arises. I would posit that the conflict has little to do with the perception of perdurance and instead, a substrate of fear: fear of being known completely and fully being rejected. Intimacy then serves as a means of awareness which lies beyond the individual and is extended to that one who has entered the dance as a life-long partner. Self-preservation no longer means the preservation of the self in context to the individual, but regarding that individual which has entered the dance of life with you. Self-preservation, at this point, becomes more aligned with a sense of self-sacrifice for the continuation of the other, to the point that neither have need to ask, "What is in it for me?" Instead, they are freed to the chaotic joy of learning what is in it for the other. Make no mistake, those you love most dearly you will wound, the question is not how do I not wound them, it is not how do I avoid being wounded, it is instead; how do I care for the wounds that I cause. Is it possible that in the midst of wounding those with which we share this beautiful dance, that we may deepen intimacy? The answer is simply: yes. Can you take ownership and in the midst of guilt, recognize that there is no need for shame? Can you embrace your failures with honest remorse and create room for the chaos of wounding? Order would tell us to fix the problem and move on, either in defense of the action or abandonment of the partner. Chaos would push toward blame and rage. Balance, however, would open the door for both to fault, both to hurt, both to heal, and both to build trust and intimacy in the midst of the chaos.

The anxious mind shutters at the thought of being exposed in moments of blame, instead, it would choose to blend with the shadows to run for shame. Balance, in the midst of anxiety, will push for an option between the binary pattern of fight or flight. There are no safe moments in intimacy, at best, there is the truth of being seen for the shadow and the persona that you are, and loved, in spite of the discrepancy. At its worst, it is the stumbling of the partner, the dashing of hopes, and flight to self-preservation at the cost of the other, but then, chaos and order is accepted. I find that in marriage, you have two partners, the partner that is the sum total of themselves and the partner which is the sum total of our hopes in them. It is necessary to grieve the loss of one, or you will inevitably lose the other or both. To carry both, it places expectations of hope onto the person that exists, hope that is not realistic, not true to the person with whom you have chosen to dance. To grieve the loss of that partner with whom is the sum total of your hopes is to begin to move toward a beautiful chaos of enjoying them as they are, absent of what we hope they may be.

When we dance in the dark, we dance in trust that the other knows the intricacy of the shared dance and yet, we provide the freedom for innovative moves as we have given room to our own awkwardness in the midst of change.

This is the beginning of expression in the midst of anxiety. It cannot be expressed in a vacuum as it would only serve as potential data waiting to be interpreted. Expression in a community is risk, it is not safe, and it is counter-intuitive, and goes against the instincts of self-preservation. However, it is risk that is worth the pain and disappointment as it allows for greater awareness of the self as an individual, and the self in those we love.

Part III
Expressing, Engaging, Embracing

"My music is the spiritual expression of what I am – my faith, my knowledge, my being."

— John Coltrane

Chapter 13
The Heroism of Expression

There will be moments when the bottom falls beneath your feet and words will not suffice to communicate the pain and hurt burning inside your heart. These painful realities deserve more than gracious platitudes. The anxious mind will run toward self-protection, desperately eliminating anything it cannot control. It will cling to simple, repetitive habits that offer an inkling of control. It will lead you down roads of isolation, back alleys where you will only serve as the silent shadow on a dimly lit wall.

Anxiety tells us that it is not safe to be seen or known. Yet, still, the burning heart aches to be known. This ambivalence, though it may seem only to add confusion, is the fight between the shadow and persona. It is but a small crack in the wall that separates what wants to be known from the world around it. It is the fight that says yes and no, all at the same time to the surfacing cries of the heart. The anxious mind says, "Stay quiet, hide, run," while the shadow waiting to spring with poetic angst cries, "I want to be seen, to be known and loved, only as I am – no mask, no hiding." As the mind races from extreme to extreme, the heart writhes in pain, helpless and waiting.

So many thoughts racing, so many extremes receding and ebbing in opposing direction, each serving a purpose, either to protect or to expose what lies beneath. This wild place, these wild things flow together to make something new, something greater. Wendell Berry put it in a way that is far more artistic than my feeble attempts:

The Peace of Wild Things

When despair for the world grows in me
and I wake in the night at the least sound
in fear of what my life and my children's lives may be,
I go and lie down where the wood drake
rests in his beauty on the water, and the great heron feeds.
I come into the peace of wild things
who do not tax their lives with forethought
of grief. I come into the presence of still water.
And I feel above me the day-blind stars
Waiting with their light. For a time
I rest in the grace of the world, and am free.

The anxious mind wants to run from the wild into seclusion. It wants to find safe harbor from that which it perceives to be a threat, one of immense danger. Fight or flight are the only options it knows. What if there was another? What if it were possible to create a space in the midst of the wildness, if only for a few moments; in spite of every instinct and scenario flashing before your eyes, you were to be still. This is the beginning of being known.

So often the anxious mind is defined by its environment, it lives in a state of hyper-vigilance. This means that it is active, reading every expression, subtle body language, and tone in the room. There is no place to make a true impression; rather, it is only the place to react to what is perceived. It is utter loneliness. The anxious mind can perceive more information in a moment than most could in days. It is out of a perceived necessity that this occurs. It is a survival skill that is developed after layers of trauma have left their mark. It is hardwired to seek the negative perspectives, things that can be perceived as threats. It is not meant for expression, rather, it is meant for preparation. It is prepared to confront or flee, but not to be known. Being known, at this moment, would mean that the anxious mind would be vulnerable. It would be seen as it is, scared and cringing at the fear of being overtaken.

Just as the Persona and the Shadow sway in the tension of an awkward dance, so does the anxious mind. Just as one desires to stay and be known, the other builds facades which communicate acceptability, while it seeks to be seen as the mess it is, so it is with the anxious mind. Somewhere, between the extremes of fight and flight, there is space to lay down in the wild places. There is a place of tension that exists, a third option if you will, that says stay, just stay. That third option is what undoes the anxious mind. It is not fight nor is it flight, it is simply: be still, be aware that this moment contains more than our fearful reactions perceive. It does not mean control the anxious thoughts; it does not mean stop worrying, for this will happen even in the midst of stillness.

It means that choices, which were not available to the anxious mind, are now present. It means that over time, awareness will develop and in the midst of this awareness, there will be space for the mind to begin to struggle with calmness. This requires repetition and patience. You will fail and struggle, and you will still experience anxiety. It is the beginning of the journey.

As has been said before, the Shadow seeks to express itself. It is the part of every person that holds both chaos and that which has not been tamed by the Persona. It is the great wilderness of the soul, that which holds the depth of our passions and our deepest secrets. When the Shadow is suppressed the most, anxiety will be at its highest. This means that the internal battle is not being known and loved, rather, a fear of being known and rejected. The fear of rejection and abandonment are the hallmarks of many disorders and if left unchecked, causes such damage. This is because it tells the individual that they are inherently bad, worthless, and unlovable. It is the voice of shame overriding the basic needs of the individual, depriving them of community, perdurance, continuation, and pattern.

Nonetheless, it begs the question; why is shame so powerful? Why is it that so many take healthy guilt and turn it into self-loathing? Guilt, in the proper context, is a necessary part of human existence. It is that which reminds us that we have stepped beyond a norm or moral threshold and yet, it seems inherent, in most, to translate this beyond its intended point. If one says that I have done a bad thing, it does not mean that I am a bad person. Rather, I would say that it communicates much the opposite. The fact that guilt within an individual shows a recognition, that a behavior or action is a break from their own personal norm, in other words, when one feels guilt, it means that they are healthy. It is much more concerning when a sense of healthy guilt does not exist.

However, when shame is what is concluded from guilt, self-hatred becomes the cell in which the heart resides. Shame says that there is no room for expression, as any expression from a bad person must be intrinsically bad. Yet, it is expression which draws back to community, perdurance, pattern, and continuation. Honest expression is the freedom to say that though one may have faults, they are not worthless, much the opposite. Acknowledging the darkness that exists within, empowers and emboldens the individual to move forward. It finally admits that there is a reality to the darkness and chaos within and that it is not bad or good, rather, it just is. Over the years, I have found that shame has robbed me of many joys. As a survivor of abuse, I was taught that I am a burden that had to be tolerated. I remember with great clarity the screams, "I hate you! I wish you had never been born! I am going to kill you!" Those words did more damage to the heart of a young boy than all the physical abuse combined. I believed those words and in some ways, still struggle not to. They are always there, just in the back of my mind, waiting, waiting for just the right moment, when I do or say the wrong thing, "You are worthless!" The echoes ring through my soul and panic ensues. It was the language that I was taught, it was the language that has, at times, motivated me to accomplish many things, but at what cost? It was the power of abusive expression that led me down a dark path for many years. It was this expression that taught me that any expression I might show is already lacking, somehow fundamentally flawed, as it flowed from a fundamentally flawed person.

It is true that we are fundamentally flawed, everyone is. The danger is when it becomes an isolated statement. When one says that I am uniquely damaged in a way that no one can understand, love, or embrace. This is the chaos of self-hatred and yet, as much power as it has to subdue the heart in shame, it has the same power to free the heart from it.

Marriage 101

A couple came for marriage counseling. For the sake of anonymity, we will call them Anna and John. Anna had begged John to seek therapy for years. She knew that something was wrong with their marriage and her initial response was to reach out for help. She had asked friends and family for advice. She was told on many occasions that, "This is just how men are." This was followed with a list of descriptors such as lazy, thoughtless, immature, childish, etc. John was a man in his mid-thirties. He and his wife were both professionals and worked very hard to make a successful home. John often worked long hours. He would return home exhausted and many times, irritable. He had a room which he called his 'man cave.' It was equipped with a refrigerator, a computer, a large-screen television, and an old, worn-out couch that Anna would not allow to be placed anywhere else in the house. It was a remnant from John's bachelor days. The 'man cave' was a grown man's version of a tree house. There was one rule that John maintained with his cave, 'No girls allowed.' Yes, Anna was not allowed in the 'man cave.' It was not as though Anna was begging to get in, but for John, it was clear a 'man cave' is only that as long as there is only a man in it. Over time, John began to spend more of his evenings hiding away in his room, mostly playing whatever videogame was popular at the moment. He was online, talking to people all over the world. They would meet at the same time every night online, and would play later and later each night. When I asked John what drew him to this virtual world, his response would shape the context of the next several sessions. "I go in there because I can escape. I can take out my frustrations, and my friends respect me. I'm good at gaming; I mean, really good. I get to be the popular guy, you know?"

I asked with more depth about what it meant to be seen as the 'popular guy,' and if there were other places he felt popular. "No, man, I mean, at work, I get a ton of crap from my boss. When I come home, my wife is always on me about not doing stuff. It's like nothing I do is good enough. I tried for a long time to get it right, but I finally just gave up. That's why I have my own space; it can be messy, and I don't have to hear how filthy it is or how this or that thing isn't done or right, or whatever."

We were not talking about being popular, we were talking about being enough. Session after session, John and I met one on one. We talked about his childhood. His father was an alcoholic, often critical of John. He wanted John to play baseball. John was more artistic in nature; there was little interest in competitive sports. John's mother was often tired. She worked two different jobs and was the primary provider for the family. John's father was often unemployed, shifting from one job to another. Though he spent a lot of time at home, he was often drunk and according to John, "He was an angry drunk."

John described his time in high school as being awkward. He was a big fan of comic books and loved superheroes. He would often spend time writing his own comics in which he was the hero. He would pursue evil villains and save the day. John was extremely creative, and this was something that his father could not relate. John described one argument which stood out vividly in his mind: "John, why the hell do you waste your time with this garbage? Drawing and writing stories, this is what you do? When your mom was pregnant, all I wanted was a son, and then we had you. I'm still waiting for a son, not some pansy that sits and doodles on notebooks. We should have just named you Jane, at least it would have fit you."

It was, at this moment, that tears broke through John's pensive stare. There it was; the shadow had emerged. He was tangible for the first time in years. He was open, still hurting and broken, just as his father had left him so many years before.

Toward the end of the session, I asked John if he still drew comics. He laughed, "I gave that stuff up a long time ago. I guess my dad was right, it was a waste of time." I asked him if he would be willing to try it one more time. His eyes awkwardly lit up. He left the office and continued his week. When he arrived for the next session, he had a small binder with him. He held it with a delicate and secure grip. The session began, and he opened the binder, "I tried my best, but I'm pretty rusty. I hope it makes some sense, probably doesn't, but it's all I could come up with." I moved my chair forward and asked John to go through the story with me. It was about a boy who was born in a dysfunctional family. When the boy was twelve, he found an old cave in a mountain close to his home. Inside the cave was a long staff, it was gold with an iridescent quality. The boy walked cautiously toward the staff, amazed by its beauty. He picked it up and when he did, the staff glowed brightly and engulfed the whole chamber in light. He fell unconscious, and when he awoke, he found himself levitating above the ground. He soon discovered that the staff had granted him great strength as well. He returned home quietly, entering his house as it was late. His father was waiting, and as soon he saw the boy, he began to yell. The yelling grew louder, and the boy's mother tried to calm him. Blinded by rage, he struck her down. She fell to the floor, grasping her arm in pain. The boy, remembering the powers that he now had, stepped forward to defend his mother and with one swift punch, sent his father flying across the room. The boy would go on to save the world time and time again, and the father never hit or even shouted from that day forward.

John finished the story and looked nervously at me. "How...how was it? I mean, I guess it sounds pretty stupid and all, and the artwork is horrible."

"John," I said, "it is absolutely amazing! This is your story! You are that boy, your power was your creativity, and you survived your father's wrath. This creativity gave you a voice; it gave you strength and that hero is you! John, I am so proud of you."

John's reaction was skeptical, "Man, this is what therapists are supposed to say, right? You're great; you can do it, you're special, that kind of stuff, it's part of your job. I don't mean to be disrespectful or anything, but I just don't believe you."

"John," I replied, "whose pen wrote the story? Whose hand drew the pictures? You're telling me that you're the hero of your story, I'm just putting in different words. Can I tell you what impressed me the most? It was the risk you took in drawing and telling this story. You took something that was used to shame you, by your own father nonetheless, you took it up, engaged yourself fully, and then showed such bravery in bringing it into the session. John, I am truly proud of you."

Over the next few weeks, we began to work out ways of risking in other areas. John began to become more aware that his wife's concerns were not because of his failure, rather, because she believed that he was capable of being the man she saw in him.

Finally, it was time to resume couple's therapy. John was more receptive to his wife's perspective. He began to come up with solutions which involved risk. He began showing more affection, not because it was expected, but rather, because he felt the freedom. He used his creativity in the arts to make love notes for his wife, often depicting her as a hero in her own right. He explained that she was his hero. He became aware of the patience and commitment that she had shown and understood the strength that it took. Roughly six months later, John and Anna attended what would be their last session. I will never forget the words that came from this now-impassioned couple.

When the session started, Anna spoke up, "Jason, we have big news, big news!" Her eyes began to tear up, "Three days ago, I came home from work and John was in his 'man cave.' My first thought was, *seriously? Still this?* I thought he was withdrawing again. So I broke the big 'no girls' rule and threw open the door. I was ready to really let him have a piece of my mind! Then I saw him. Jason, he wasn't on his computer, he wasn't chatting in some game. He was painting the room. He had moved that disgusting couch out; there was now a crib in its place. He was making a nursery. Jason, I promise, I didn't tell him to get rid of his 'man cave,' I never mentioned anything about it, but there he was, turning it into a nursery. Which is the other big news, we are having a baby."

I looked at John, "The man cave? Really? You got rid of it? What made you think of this?" John looked me in the eyes, strong, confident, and yet, caring. "Jason, every boy needs a hero. I learned from you that it is supposed to be his dad or mom. They weren't there so, for years, I had to make up my heroes. I wasn't pretending to have heroes. I was pretending to have a dad. I never had anyone take my art seriously! No one ever told me that they were proud of me being who I am just because of who I am. I know you are not my dad, but you were the man that helped me see that I could do it! I can do it! I am just figuring it out. I mean, I'm just figuring out how to love Anna. When she cries, I don't feel shame; I don't feel burdened, I feel, well, I feel love for her. I am figuring out how to be the husband that my dad never was; I will be the father that my son needs. I will be his hero, no matter what it takes. This stuff used to freak me out, you know? I remember to have these panic attacks when Anna would talk about therapy but Anna was right, I needed help. I can do this! Jason, we don't need therapy anymore." It was with this proclamation that John stood up, crossing the span between us, and hugged me. It wasn't the kind of hug that a boy gives his dad. It was the kind of hug that a man gives because he is confident enough to express his heart. It was strong and tender; it was the hug of a hero.

I congratulated them both on the news of their baby and the birth of their newfound love. John was the hero of his story. He always was. He tried to find himself in the empty shell of a broken and battered father, but it wasn't until he could embrace the true nature of his shadow and let it be known as it was that he could see the hero that he already had become.

Everyone, anxious or otherwise, is always in the process of becoming. The process of becoming requires the risky expression of intimacy, true and honest expression. It is only in the midst of facing the fear of what we might be that we can begin to embrace that which we are.

The anxious mind will lead to escape, withdrawal, and isolation, but the tension between the shadow and the persona is that which is known and expressed in its fullness as it is.

Chapter 14
The Art of Engaging

The anxious mind works in a vicious circle, it will dread that which triggers anxiety and try to avoid it as long as possible. Then, only when it is no longer possible to avoid, it will engage with force and fury. This, in turn, creates a more traumatic sense of the trigger and the cycle intensifies. As the intensity continues, the urge to eliminate triggers becomes stronger. This constant elimination creates greater restriction on daily tasks and freedoms. Allowed to continue, this can lead to phobias such as agoraphobia.

Most individuals tend to avoid crowded places such as malls, supermarkets, or social events such as parties or sporting events. The mind adapts to the changes and continues the restrictive tendencies. This is due to the fact that while anxiety may be triggered by an external factor, it is not the underlying cause. This is why many treatments surrounding triggers are not always effective.

The underlying causation of anxiety has more to do with a sense of control, more specifically a sense, that there is a loss of control, whether partially or completely. This is why the mind avoids triggers; it is simply a way of reestablishing a sense of control in a given situation. A sense of control is just that, a sense. While an individual may exhibit control to a certain degree over an object or situation, the concept of control is much more complex. Control in the context of action, for example, may be exhibited in a simple manner such as a choice of clothing or music. While for the most part, few would give much thought to the limitation of control in either of these areas, it is important to note that with very little effort, it can be limited. For example, one may choose to listen to jazz and thus, there is a sense of control, however, the choice of music is lost should there be a loss of power, and thus, the sense of control is lost. This may seem to be a slight issue, but when multiplied with the multitude of options for the exertion of control, there is always antithetical pairing. Thus, control, even in the simplest form, functions more as a construct of the mind which encourages action. The mind adapts to options and hence, establishes the construct of consistency through action. This will be maintained until the construct is impeded, therefore establishing a break in the consistency, and thus, a break in the sense of control. This, for the most part, goes unnoticed or may present as mild frustration but when the construct of control is challenged on a foundational level, such as the perception of survival, any option can serve as a trigger. Thus, it is of great importance for the anxious mind to contemplate the utter fragility of control as a sense of safety.

There are many approaches to anxiety which target the ability to regain this sense of control, but the effectiveness of any approach will be limited to how one defines control. If control and safety are conjoined synonymously, then the mind will continue to seek control through the elimination of triggers. Thus, the continuous cycle of elimination is reinforced, and the intended outcome is not only missed, but rather, another extreme is established. It is the vacillation between these extremes, which if perceived as control, that causes the physical response of anxiety.

This begs the question; if one cannot control, with any certainty, the simplest of constructs, then why does any pursuit of control become detrimental? The answer is, if the focus is on the pursuit of control then, by all means, it will become detrimental.

However, if one begins to redefine control, not as a pursuit but rather as an experiential construct, then one gains the freedom to let go of the burden, an old model of control, and begins to gain a sense of awareness that all things are in flux at all times. This allows the anxious mind to embrace change as a norm rather than a disruption from a norm.

The adoption of control, through experience, offers a sense of control, through the ultimate reduction of responsibility, to control an environment, and clarifies the limitations of the individual's ability to control.

This means, in short, that the anxious mind will adapt more toward a sense of finite balance in the midst of vacillations between extremes, and ultimately, will attribute less importance to enforce direct change, as opposed to the acceptance of change. This will lead the individual to a construct that is less anxiety-ridden and more attuned to adaption, both emotionally and physically.

When working with clients suffering from anxiety and panic attacks, I often give a checklist of all the symptoms one would experience during a panic attack. I explain each symptom and the biological purpose it serves. Through the course of treatment, I advise them to check each symptom on the list as they experience it. As they review the list, regularly checking symptoms, they are beginning to normalize the experience. Frequently, the client will begin to expect the symptom with less and less anxiety and eventually, the symptoms themselves will diminish, as well as the overall panic attack. This approach again, is not involved in trying to control the symptoms, rather it is merely introducing a sense of order to what is perceived as a chaotic experience. The checklist itself serves to chart the frequency of symptoms. Several clients have returned to sessions with a sense of interest bordering on excitement when they have begun to understand a predominant symptom. This shift in understanding engages the individual in evaluating themselves and deepening their awareness. There is no point in which a client is instructed to try to control their panic. This would serve as a means of control that would eventually serve to increase anxiety, as the expectation would be to change a biological process that has already begun before it is even perceived.

One client, we will refer to as Jim for the sake of anonymity, came seeking treatment for anxiety. During the first session, Jim described a long history of worry mixed with bouts of depression. Jim had a long history of unhealthy relationships. He explained that many of these relationships were, "...disappointing and frustrating. When I meet someone, my mind immediately begins to race with a thousand questions in like a second. Is she fake? Is she selfish? I just don't, you know, want to get hurt. I can't stand the rejection, it makes me think I'm going to be alone for the rest of my life! I mean, what if I never meet, you know, the one? I don't want to be one of those old guys that just sits on the porch, yelling at the neighbor's kids, like, 'Hey, get off my grass!' I don't want to be that way. Maybe that's why I, you know, freak out." I asked Jim to describe his most recent relationships. "She was kind of cool, I guess. We had fun hanging out, and she liked to play Call of Duty. She wasn't, like, on her phone all the time, but...there's always a but... She wanted to move so damn fast! We were together, like, a month, you know, and she wanted to move in. I was all like, are you kidding me? Move in? Then, I freaked, I mean, on the inside, I just shut down on the outside. I didn't text or call as much because she would always bring it up. I started getting, you know, smothered. I finally just messaged her and said I couldn't do this anymore. I can't keep on dodging all these questions about moving in and marriage and the future and stuff like that. She didn't reply, you know? She just blocked me. I tried several times to talk to her and she just shut me out of her life completely."

Jim wanted intimacy, and yet, when confronted by someone who wanted the same, it created a lot of ambivalence. I asked Jim to list one person that truly knew him, the good, the bad, and the ugly. Jim paused for a short time, then, looking down to the floor, he said, "Man, I don't think anyone knows that stuff. Why would I give up that kind of info? Do you know what they could do with it if they got mad at me? They would throw every bit of it right in my face and I don't want all that drama. I mean, I tell my friends about girls or work but personal stuff, man, well, that's personal."

I asked Jim if he felt like his fear of keeping personal information inside helped him or hurt him when it came to intimacy. "Man, it totally helps. I mean, I don't want people to, you know, think I'm some weirdo or something. It's just part of life, you know? Like, my mom would always say you don't talk about politics or religion because everyone will get offended. It's just embarrassing, and I don't want to look like I don't have it all together like I'm crazy or something."

"Jim," I said, "everyone is a mess on the inside. Everyone who walks into a therapist's office thinks that they are somehow uniquely messed up. The reality is that we are all a mess and part of intimacy is letting someone experience your mess with you. It means that you are known, truly known, and loved just as you are, both good and bad, and in turn, you experience their chaos, their mess, and over time, you learn to create a new order between your messes. It is order that lets you be you, always learning, always growing, and always growing in awareness of yourself and your partner." Needless to say, Jim was not convinced, and I was glad that he had the confidence to say it. I asked him to take the week to think about the old man on the porch. I asked him to think about how many people truly knew him and what the process of becoming that man would involve.

The next week, Jim came to my office, smiling, "Jason, I thought about it and man, I get it, it scared the crap out of me, but I get it. Truth is, I get it, but I don't want to do it. Maybe it's like, I don't know how to do it. Do I just, like, walk up to a girl and say, 'Hi! I'm Jim, and I'm a mess! Want to get lunch sometime?'"

"Jim," I said, "I love your courage, and that scenario would scare just about anyone. Maybe there's another way of going about this. If you are walking up to someone and announcing that you are a mess, it might come off less as being open and more as confrontational. What if you were talking to someone about a topic that you enjoy, let's say photography, for example. Perhaps you could share why you like taking pictures of nature. I remember that you mentioned you like to take pictures of animals in nature. What is it that you find inspiring about animals in nature?"

Jim smiled, "Man, they are so majestic, like eagles, I love eagles! When I see them flying, it's like I want to spread my wings and fly with them. I just feel really free, you know? When I take a picture of an eagle, it's like I'm capturing more than the image, it's like I'm taking a picture of myself if I could fly." Jim's answer was moving in itself. I felt like I knew him a little more.

I said, "Jim, you nailed it, buddy! You told me a place in your life that makes you feel free. This is a good first step in a conversation."

"You mean, I can just talk about the things that I love and ask questions about what they love too?"

"Jim, what you shared just now with me gave me a glimpse of a part of you that I wouldn't have known, not just that you love pictures, but that you see yourself soaring with the eagles and it is how you see freedom. The old man on the porch would never tell me about that, would he?"

Jim shook his head and said, "I guess, he probably wouldn't. He would be more worried about why you're in his yard."

"Exactly! If you are sharing those things with me, it means you have invited me into your yard, your personal space. It may not be in your living room, and that's okay!"

Jim had initially ended relationships when they became too intimate. It was an attempt at control. When we tried an intimate approach, he shifted to confrontational information, which was another attempt at control and would inevitably end in the same isolation. When Jim stepped away from control to the passion, he was excited to share in ways that were invitations to intimacy. It was less trying to do it the right way and more engaging his passion, sharing his shadow. Over the course of several months, we addressed these issues with more depth, and his comfort level increased. His worry concerning loneliness abated as he was actually spending more time doing the things that he loved. He joined a community group for photographers. He would come to sessions with photos, overflowing with stories and experiences. After a few trips with the group, Jim's photos began to change. There were many shots of eagles and even a bear, but then there were photos of Jim with the group. He was smiling, and his arms were raised in one photo. I asked him about this particular photo.

Jim smiled and said, "These are my bros! That's Tom, Mike, Denise, and, of course, that's me, with my wings spread just like the eagles."

No truer words had ever been said. Jim had truly spread his wings. He was engaging wholeheartedly in the expression of his passions. In the midst of it all, he found his wings; there they were, right there in the picture, arms spread wide, soaring. Needless to say, Jim's anxiety began to decrease as he was engaging with people, including one person, in particular, Denise.

A few months after we finished therapy, I received a phone call, "Jason! It's your eagle guy, Jim! I need to book a session. We want to do pre-marriage counseling."

I responded rather excitedly, "We? Pre-marital? What? Who is this guy? Of course, I can't wait to sit with you both!" And we did.

This is the powerful side of change. It doesn't flow from new ways of trying to control the same thing. It comes with risk, it comes with adventure and passion, and of course, it comes with the individual who is constantly coming into being and accepting both the good and bad.

Chapter 15
The Great Embrace

Throughout this book, we have discussed anxiety as fear of losing control of central pieces of existence: perdurance, community, pattern, and groundedness. These terms are the basic D.N.A. of security, both for the developing child, as well as the adult. When one begins to gain a sense of awareness of self and others, each of the central pieces is challenged and changed into something new, something deeper.

This is the Necessary Struggle that Jung refers to, and it is the Necessary Struggle that every individual must face.

There are always tips and strategies for any struggle or problem, but there is only one way to embrace the Necessary Struggle, and that is to struggle. It is not elegant, it is, by nature, not an easy journey, and yet, we must first begin with the principle of awareness.

When a baby is born, there is something inherently special that happens, something that is counter-intuitive to a basic survival instinct; the baby cries. There, in the first few moments of life, breathing their first breath of air, feeling the coolness of a hospital room, being held by a doctor, a human, something that it can, by no means, conceive. The baby is vulnerable and naked, and its first response is to communicate. This would suggest that even in the midst of the unknown world, with no social learning, that the need for embrace is hardwired into this newborn. A baby is born crying for something, something that it does not yet even know and yet, when there is embrace, the initial embrace of the mother, a bond is formed. It is locked into the mind of both the mother and her baby. There is no language that a newborn could use to communicate this bond and yet, it is there. It is through growth and development that we are taught to fear, and the fear is necessary. It is that which tells us that there is more and yet, that it cannot be contrived through clever disciplines or simply working harder. No, this is something that is suggestive of the newborn's experience, as we are constantly coming into being, we are constantly born into new experiences, new environments, and new levels of social engagement. The more we learn, the more we know that there is more to learn and this is a danger to the construct of control. If we were to learn from the newborn one lesson, it might be this: when exposed, terrified, overwhelmed by a new world, it is time to breathe, express, engage that which is not yet known and find the great embrace. The great embrace is that experiential moment when comfort is found in the midst of chaos and order. It is an embrace that will be repeated with each new struggle; the embrace that tells us that our order is another's chaos. We are cold, naked, anxious, and afraid; it is the engagement which leads to the embrace in the midst of experiencing the vacillation between chaos and order on the road to intimacy.

Oscar Wilde's, *The Picture of Dorian Gray,* depicts a young man who in the height of his youth and vigor chose to embrace the path of one who does not change. He chose, in our terms, the life of the Persona, as the Shadow was stowed safely away behind locked doors. Dorian appeared unchanged throughout his life. His youth never left him, his charm ever present, but the shadow that which he hid most deeply, as if it were seen as it was, all of Dorian's mistakes, crimes, wickedness, and hatred would be evident to the viewer. Much later in the book, Basil, the painter of Dorian Gray's picture, returns for one last look at his opus. Dorian takes Basil to the room where the picture has been locked, unveils the painting, and in a fit of rage, kills Basil. It is then still enraged that he turns the knife toward the painting, The Shadow plunges the knife through the canvas, thus inflicting the wound to his own body. As Dorian lay dying, every blemish, mark, and scar appeared on Dorian. Finally, in his rage to destroy that which he hated, Dorian was indeed only wounding himself. One cannot separate the Persona from the Shadow, just as one cannot separate light from the flame. These are acts of control based on only a portion of the greater fabric of the Necessary Struggle. As it was true with Dorian, it is true with each and every individual. That which we seek to hide the most will find its way to the surface. If it is repressed with violent ire, it will erupt forth with the same violence with which it had been repressed. If it is embraced as it is, if it is offered up in the delicate nature of intimacy, it will arise gently and as delicately as the intimacy itself. It cannot be solved, outwitted, or neglected, for it is as much of the individual being as the Persona. Though shrouded in shame, this component has the keys to creativity, depth, warmth, and a counter-intuition that may, at times, upend the persona, but will over time, balance with growth.

Carl Jung viewed it as follows: "The greatest and most important problems in life are fundamentally insoluble. They can never be solved but only outgrown."

If it's possible for an individual to know the darkness within and to embrace the condition of the darkness, it is only then that they may be able to embrace the darkness of others. The darkness that is chaos to one is merely order to another.

Growth is fraught with pain; it is the experience of the mystery of this pain which removes the deeper truths and awareness, like a flower in early spring arises from the cold darkness to express its true beauty.

The anxious mind is infatuated with the false sense of control that, for a time, had served a self-soothing purpose. It is when one's awareness exceeds the limits of this self-soothing that anxiety spirals to greater heights. This is not a sign of weakness, nor is it a sign of insanity, rather to the contrary, it is merely the pangs of birth. Hence, we emerge, no longer comforted by the womb of control that no longer could contain us. The anxious mind is a marker on the path of the Necessary Struggle, it is not the threat that the mind perceives.

This is not about good or bad, right or wrong, neither is about safe or unsafe, it is merely awareness of what is unknown. Shame will tell you that you are beyond help, that you are bad and hopeless, that you are not safe and yet, shame also is a womb that must be outgrown. For one to be good does not, by necessity, define them as safe. As a matter of fact, it is that which is good, that which is aware and growing in true honesty that is the most dangerous to those who hide in the dark.

C.S. Lewis in *The Lion the Witch and the Wardrobe,* says as much in the discussion between Lucy and Mr. Beaver. She cannot conceive of Aslan as he is beyond her conception.

"…if there's anyone who can appear before Aslan without their knees knocking, they're either braver than most or else just silly."

"Then he isn't safe?" said Lucy.

"Safe," said Mr. Beaver. "Don't you hear what Mrs. Beaver tells you? Who said anything about safe? 'Course he isn't safe. But he's good."

He isn't safe, but he is good. This is such an echo of the anxious mind in growth. The Great Embrace is not safe, it is counter-intuitive, and, in many ways much like Aslan, it contains an element of self-sacrifice.

Growth is, in essence, the sacrifice of the old self, the old womb for that which is constantly coming into being. It is only in this journey that we find the balance between the extremes, and it is here that we will continually find the greater balance. It is the embrace of the true self, both Shadow and Persona. It is the Great Embrace in the midst of Quiet Chaos.